What You Need to Know about Dementia

What You Need to Know about Dementia

Selva Sugunendran

To order additional copies of this book, contact:
Xlibris
1-888-795-4274
www.Xlibris.com
Orders@Xlibris.com
769488

Dedication

This book is dedicated to Jeevachandran,
his loving wife Saro and family.

Contents

Introduction...xi

Acknowledgements xv

Chapter 1   History of Alzheimer's Disease 1

Chapter 2   What is Dementia?...7

Chapter 3   Types of Dementia 16

Chapter 4   Causes and Diagnosis of Dementia....................30

Chapter 5   Stages of Alzheimer's Disease.........................54

Chapter 6   Importance of Clinical Evaluation 59

Chapter 7   Prevention of Alzheimer's Disease 62

Chapter 8   Treatment of Alzheimer's Disease 75

Chapter 9   Powerful Natural Remedies for Dementia and
             Alzheimer's...92

Chapter 10   Coping with the Signs and Symptoms 109

Chapter 11   Preventing and Slowing the Progression of
             Dementia 116

Chapter 12   Providing Successful Dementia Therapy.............135

Chapter 13   Keep Dementia at Bay 142

Chapter 14   Prediction of Disease Spread with MRI Scans 148

Chapter 15   How Brain Building Can Help Delay
             Alzheimer's and Dementia............................. 151

Chapter 16   How to Become a Successful Alzheimer's
             Disease Caregiver 157

Chapter 17   A Guide to Homecare 176

Chapter 18   Future Dementia Treatments and Cure................187

Conclusions...201

Contents

1. Who may be affected by Alzheimer's disease?................205
2. Signs & Symptoms of Alzheimer's disease 207
3. Understanding signs and symptoms of Alzheimer's disease..209
4. What actually happens to the brain over time when Alzheimer's disease progresses...............................211
5. Communicating with your doctor about your Alzheimer's disease 213
6. Diagnosing Alzheimer's disease................................215
7. Preparing for the future during progression of Alzheimer's disease 217
8. The future outlook for Alzheimer's patients 219
9. Preventing Alzheimer's disease 221
10. Understanding Vascular Dementia 223
11. Dementia with Lewy bodies 225
12. Understanding Frontotemporal Dementia.....................227
13. Dementia is a progressive disease..............................229
14. Getting dementia help and advice in the UK...............231
15. Guidelines for advanced stages of dementia..................233
16. How Dementia Progresses and the Stages of the Mental Decline..235
17. How to improve healthcare for those affected by Dementia..238
18. In search of dementia treatment................................240
19. Stress and how it damages the brain..........................242
20. Understanding signs and symptoms of Alzheimer's disease..244

21. The survival trends for people with dementia....................246
22. Understanding Diagnosis and Treatment of Dementia 248
23. Assessment & Planning Of Care for those affected by Dementia 250
24. How can you take care of a person with Dementia? 252
25. Looking after a patient with dementia 254
26. The importance of palliative care for dementia 256
27. The impact of dementia worldwide in 2015 258
28. Important facts about dementia in 2016 260
29. Possible trend shifts in the future of dementia incidence...262
30. The global cost of dementia treatment 264

INTRODUCTION

"**W**HAT YOU NEED to know about Dementia" aims to demystify the oft-misunderstood term for loss of cognitive ability and how it impacts the lives of those who are diagnosed and their families. Told in an easy to understand format, this guide walks you through a process no one asks to be a part of, but unfortunately, many will find themselves facing head on.

Dementia, in its very basic form, is the gradual loss of cognitive function that affects all aspects of daily living like loss of short-term memory, dysphagia, incontinence, declining communication skills, behavioral issues, in addition to many other symptoms.

For those who suffer from any of the varied types of dementia and those who care for them, it is a life-altering diagnosis that they struggle daily to understand, control, and fear that one day they'll be diagnosed with.

Inside the pages of this comprehensive guide, you'll learn all the nuances of this incurable, yet often minimally treatable disease. From the early signs and symptoms through to each of the more impactful stages of this disease and how it impacts lives, affects psychosocial skills, and impairs otherwise healthy individuals from all walks of life, you'll walk away with a better understanding of the disease's process and will feel a sense of empowerment to face whatever may come next in your life or in the lives of those you love.

A peek inside the front cover of this book will assure you that all the answers to your questions or answers to questions you might not have ever thought to ask will be answered. Beginning with an easy-to-understand definition of dementia to how to acquire a diagnosis and what to do after you've received a diagnosis, there's no stone unturned from Step A to Step B and beyond.

With so many different types of dementia, it can be difficult for lay people to understand where to begin a search for information. This book gathers all that information in one place and lays it out for you to mull over, write down, or perhaps take to your clinician for further discussion.

After a diagnosis, you might not know what step to take first. After all, no one anticipates that they'll receive news that they are in fact experiencing symptoms of cognitive loss. How, then, does one proceed?

Management of the disease and the appointments, treatments, and lifestyle changes that accompany it can be overwhelming. That's precisely why this book was written, to take the confusion and sudden feeling of loss out of the process, or at least lessen its impact on the diagnosed individual and their loved ones.

In addition to learning about what happens following a diagnosis, you'll learn all the risk factors involved and how they might impact your life. You may not know that some of the risk factors can be modified to lessen the likelihood of a diagnosis for you.

An aspect of dementia and its care you might not have considered or heard about before is aromatherapy. Aromatherapy has shown promise in managing symptoms that are often associated with dementia like anxiety, disorientation, frustration, and depression in randomized controlled patient trials.

Beyond treatments from those who suffer from this disease, you'll also learn the top ten things that every dementia caregiver needs to remember to help them cope with the worsening symptoms of memory loss and physical decline. As with any other illness, those caring for people with this disease often suffer extreme fatigue, regret, guilt, and sadness. That is to be expected, but that too should be monitored. Healthy outlets are necessary. This book details some proven ideas to help you get through the more difficult part of the process.

Dementia aids and products can also help ease some of the burden caregivers might bear. You'll find information about some of them and how they might fit into your treatment plan, and discover key steps that may help you to provide successful dementia therapy at home.

No matter what stage of the process you and your family find yourself in, this timely, informational guide can help ease your mind, give you some points to think about, and help you to make the best choices possible for the one you love.

ACKNOWLEDGEMENTS

DURING THE LAST 12 to 15 months of active research into Dementia and while following a University diploma course on Dementia, my knowledge was enriched by so many people, who have given their time, their research, experiences, opinions and wisdom.

Unfortunately there is not enough room here to acknowledge each and every one of them. My special heartful thanks go to all those kind people.

Thanks are also due to my family for their support and understanding as I spent long hours while researching and travelling to gather the data required to write this book.

My thanks go to my mother for instilling in me the importance of prevention over treatment and my father for teaching the disciplines necessary to take on and be successful in any challenge I undertook. I would also acknowledge my grandmother for instilling in me the

Christian values of loving, caring and sharing, in addition to learning to protect my honesty and my integrity at all times. These have become my core values and belief.

I was so impressed by the questions my grandson Jason (aged 10) and my grandaughter Lisa (aged 7) asked me about current research and why we have not found a way of preventing Dementia after 115 years or so. Their questions were centered on the 40% of cost of Dementia being borne by Informal care (unpaid care provided by family and others). I believe that there are many more young people who would grow up to do something to raise funds and accelerate the research into methods of early detection and prevention of Dementia.

Many thanks also go to those who have touched my life including prayer warriors Griselda Yohendran, Mark & Rumalee Ruth (Chuttie) Abraham, Ramona Devadason, Rosemary & Saverus, Jeevaraj and many others.

Finally, I would like to thank those who have inspired me including my very good friend (and source of inspiration at work) Fred Jane, as well as Pasters T.U. Thomas, Ranjit and Ernest Paul.

My heartful thanks go to all those I have mentioned above and those I couldn't mention. You know who you are!

I cannot end this acknowledgment without giving thanks to God who has provided me with everything I need as illustrated in Philippines 4: Verses 11-13

CHAPTER ONE

History of Alzheimer's Disease

ALZHEIMER'S DISEASE is named after the German psychologist, Alois Alzheimer. Whilst it is presented as a twentieth century disease, the brain degeneration, cognitive impairment and disturbing behavioral and psychiatric problems which characterize the disease have most likely been around for centuries.

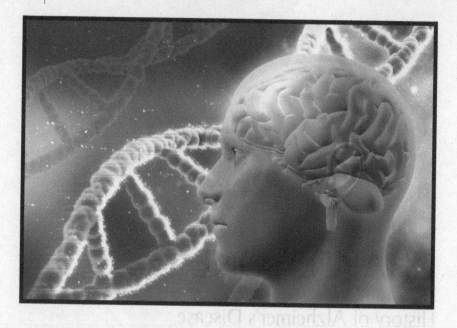

While Dr. Alzheimer is the disease's namesake, Alzheimer's colleague, Emil Kraepelin, played an equally important role in the identification of the disease.

Kraepelin isolated and grouped together the symptoms of the disorder, suggesting they were a unique disease process, while Alzheimer was the first to understand what was actually happening in the brains of Alzheimer's patients.

He discovered unusual plaques and tangles in the brain of one of his patients, a fifty year old woman, who exhibited the symptoms of the disorder identified by Kraepelin.

After Kraepelin and Alzheimer's identification of the disease in the early twentieth century, Alzheimer's disease history shows that not many advances were made in understanding or treating the disease.

This could have been because the disease could only be diagnosed after a patient's death: at the autopsy, until the end of the twentieth century.

Initially, the disease was diagnosed in patients between the ages of 45 and 65 and labeled as "presenile dementia." The name Alzheimer's disease only gained popularity in the 70s and 80s as a label for patients over the age of 65. Now, the disease has recognizable and diagnosable symptoms, which can appear in patients as young as 30.

Typically, an aggressive type of Alzheimer's disease that occurs in patients under the age of 65 has a known genetic factor, while the appearance of the disease in patients over 65 has a number of other factors in regards to its development, such as health, occupation, and environment.

Recent advances in science and technology have led to a promising new era in Alzheimer's disease history. Cognex, the first FDA-approved drug used to slow the disease process, hit the markets in 1990, and three others soon followed.

The medications slow-down the cognitive impairment in patients with mild to moderate Alzheimer's disease by boosting depleted levels of acetylcholine in the brain. These are crucial to the healthy functioning of neurons.

Other research is being done on ways to prevent Alzheimer's from developing further, and even preventing its onset.

Certain hormones such as estrogen and anti-inflammatory drugs such as aspirin have been found to have a mediating effect, and environmental factors, such as mentally demanding occupations, dance, and chess have been found to decrease older people's chances of developing Alzheimer's.

Even something as simple as wearing a seatbelt or helmet could be crucial to preventing Alzheimer's disease. Early detection techniques are being honed to improve treatment of the disease. For example, genetic research has discovered genetic markers for Familial (as in coming from the family: genetic) Alzheimer's disease as well as non-familial Alzheimer's.

In addition, advanced technology, such as MRIs and PET scans, are being used to detect structural changes in the brain that may indicate the development of Alzheimer's disease before symptoms even begin.

As the Baby Boomer generation begins to age, scientists fear the strain a large number of dementia patients could place upon the healthcare and social welfare systems; therefore, researchers are scrambling to make Alzheimer's disease history.

The initial symptoms of the disease are loss of the capability to form new memories and inability to recall current events. Diagnosis of Alzheimer's disease is based on cognitive tests and brain scan.

As the disease advances, the individual shows the symptoms of confusion, irritability, aggression, mood fluctuations, language problems and finally long-term memory loss.

The vivacious functions of body fail to operate and death is the decisive fate. Less than 3% percent live for about fourteen years after the diagnosis of the disease.

The precise cause of Alzheimer's disease is still not understood. Research carried out all over the world designate that the disease is caused due to the accretion of plaques and tangles in the brain. However, new research indicates that there could possibly be another underlying cause.

Although treatment for this disorder is available, the chances of complete recovery is much less. More than 500 clinical trials have been carried out but the meticulous reason for the occurrence of this disorder is yet not available.

Stimulation, balanced diet and exercise are recommended for the patients of this disorder. As Alzheimer's disease is degenerative and an incurable disease, proper management of the patient is essential. Family support is strongly required.

Who are at risk?

The prime factor to blame for Alzheimer's disease is increased age and as the age of the individual increases, the risk of this disease also increases. According to a report, about 10% of the individuals belonging to the age group of 65, and 50% of the individuals of the age group of 85 suffer from Alzheimer's disease.

According to a guesstimate, the number of patients of this disease in the world will increase to 140 million by 2050. Genetic factors are also thought to be responsible for this disease and most of the individuals develop this disorder after the age of 70.

However, about 2-5% of the individuals develop the symptoms in their early forties and fifties. The children of a person with early onset of the symptoms of Alzheimer's disease are at 50% risk of developing this disorder. The gene located on chromosome 19 (APOE e4)is believed to be responsible for this disease.

However, in the majority of cases, specific genetic risks have not been identified yet. Other risk factors associated are high blood pressure, coronary artery disease, high blood cholesterol and diabetes. All the patients of Down syndrome develop this disorder in their forties.

CHAPTER TWO

What is Dementia?

"DEMENTIA" IS A phrase which refers to a set of mental conditions like Vascular dementia, Mixed Dementia, Dementia with Lewy Bodies and Fronto-temporal Dementia. However, it is mostly associated with aging and a disease called Alzheimer's.

Dementia is loss of cognitive ability in a person, either due to global brain injury or some disease that results in memory loss. If it occurs before the age of 65, then it is known as early onset dementia. The word dementia comes from a Latin word meaning madness.

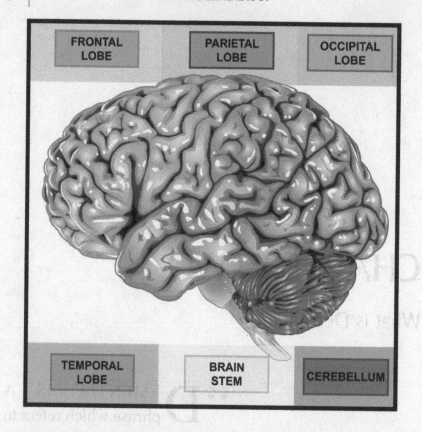

FRONTAL LOBE

PARIETAL LOBE

OCCIPITAL LOBE

TEMPORAL LOBE

BRAIN STEM

CEREBELLUM

It can be considered as a non-specific illness syndrome where the areas of the brain concerned with memory, language, attention and problem solving are severely affected. About six months are required for the disease to be diagnosed and in later stages, the affected persons may become disoriented in time.

Dementia is treatable up to a certain degree, but as the disease advances, the symptoms become incurable. The symptoms of the disease may or may not be reversible and it depends upon the etiology of the disease.

The possibility of complete freedom from the symptoms of dementia is less than 10%. Dementia can be confused with the short-term syndrome, delirium, if careful assessment of the patient's history is not done as the symptoms are somewhat similar.

Depression and psychosis can be used for differentiating dementia and delirium. Many types of dementia are known that differ slightly in their symptoms.

The symptoms of different types may overlap, so diagnosis is done by nuclear brain scanning techniques. Most common types of dementia include Alzheimer's disease, Vascular and Frontotemporal dementia and dementia with Lewy bodies. A person may suffer from one or more types of dementia simultaneously at a time.

The medical term, dementia, does not represent any one single disease. It is a term used to describe a medical condition that is characterised by a group of symptoms - symptoms that are not a normal part of the ageing process. The condition can be simplistically defined as a decline in intellectual functioning so severe that the sufferer cannot perform routine activities and tasks.

Dementia related ailments are caused by the loss of brain chemicals and the degeneration of cerebral matter which occur when brain cells become damaged and die without replacement.

That process subsequently leads to the brain retrogressing which induces a progressive loss of normal mental functions. The result is dementia. Alzheimer's disease is the most common cause of dementia although there are many other diseases that can lead to the condition.

The term, dementia, normally implies a permanent state of mental confusion as opposed to delirium which describes a temporary mental disturbance. For this reason, it is fortunate that the degenerative disease usually occurs later in life, rather than early, as it robs victims of the ability to think, remember and reason. Worst of all, the condition is irreversible.

Dementia stage has a marked deterioration of memory, impaired concentration and an increasing tendency to fatigue and anxiety. Nothing more than an obvious failure of memory may be observed for a year or two because of the relatively slow progress of the disease. There is a further deterioration, which is particularly evident around practical everyday skills.

At this stage, the home begins to take on an air of squalor as the person is no longer able to use the washing machine and the vacuum cleaner. Similar deficits occur in the workplace which leads to early retirement and all intellectual function is grossly impaired.

WHAT IS ALZHEIMER'S?

Alzheimer's is a disease that destroys brain cells, hampers communication between neurons and seriously impairs a person's ability to function. Memory, language and thought are particularly affected.

Symptoms include asking the same question over and over and getting lost in familiar places. The chances of Alzheimer's increases steadily after age 65, but it is not the mild memory decline associated with normal aging. It is a degenerative brain disease.

Alzheimer's usually starts with the symptom of memory loss. This may affect the patient's ability to learn new things, focus on tasks, and do the things that they once did in life. Many sufferers start to experience a different type of personality. The person may become depressed, angry, and may even lash out at those around them for no logical reason.

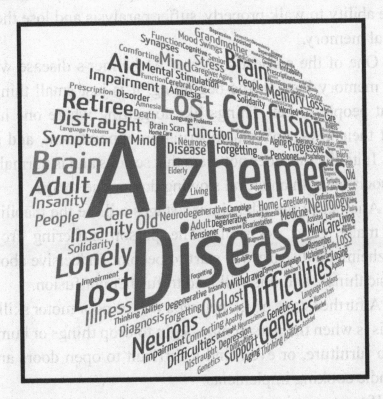

There is a progressive deterioration in both the person's mental and bodily state and ability of their recall of events. There is also a difference in the actions and personality of the person with Alzheimer's, with their ordinary actions becoming a thing of the past.

For example, someone who has always been gentle and kind may begin to use filthy words and make inappropriate sexual advances or become violent and begin striking and lashing out at people.

In the later stages of Alzheimer's, the person eventually becomes incapable of performing any task at all. They also become doubly incontinent, lose their power of speech, lose the ability to walk properly, suffer paralysis and lose their total memory.

One of the earliest stages of Alzheimer's disease will be memory loss. In the beginning, it is just small things that people forget. Things like forgetting where one has put their keys, not remembering an appointment, and so on. Initially, this does not seem that serious and is normally associated with a natural slowing down, due to age.

Another of the Alzheimer's stages will be the inability to make good decisions. The person suffering from Alzheimer's disease will start to become indecisive about basic things, and this will lead to further confusion.

A further stage of Alzheimer's will be poor motor skills. This is when the person may begin to drop things or bump into furniture, or even find it difficult to open doors and handle cooking implements.

If treatment is given early enough, it can slightly slow down the disease, but unfortunately, it is incurable at the time of writing.

Once Alzheimer's disease is diagnosed, then the person should be given as much help and aid as feasible, especially in the early stages. Unfortunately, many people who are diagnosed with Alzheimer's disease are conscious at first that something is wrong with them (although they may go into denial), and being aware you are "losing your mind" can be a truly shocking and frightening experience.

THE DIFFERENCE BETWEEN ALZHEIMER'S DISEASE AND DEMENTIA

"Dementia" is a term that has replaced a more out-of-date word, "senility," to refer to cognitive changes with advanced age.

Dementia includes a group of symptoms, the most prominent of which is memory difficulty with additional problems in at least one other area of cognitive functioning, including language, attention, problem solving, spatial skills, judgment, planning, or organization.

These cognitive problems are a noticeable change compared to the person's cognitive functioning earlier in life and are severe enough to get in the way of normal daily living, such as social and occupational activities.

A good analogy to the term dementia is "fever." Fever refers to an elevated temperature, indicating that a person is sick. But it does not give any information about what is causing the sickness.

In the same way, dementia means that there is something wrong with a person's brain, but it does not provide any information about what is causing the memory or cognitive difficulties. Dementia is not a disease; it is the clinical presentation or symptoms of a disease.

There are many possible causes of dementia. Some causes are reversible, such as certain thyroid conditions or vitamin deficiencies. If these underlying problems are identified and treated, then the dementia reverses and the person can return to normal functioning.

However, most causes of dementia are not reversible. Rather, they are degenerative diseases of the brain that get worse over time. The most common cause of dementia is AD, accounting for as many as 70-80% of all cases of dementia.

Approximately 5.3 million Americans currently live with AD. As people get older, the prevalence of AD increases, with approximately 50% of people age 85 and older having the disease.

It is important to note, however, that although AD is extremely common in later years of life, it is not part of normal aging. For that matter, dementia is not part of normal aging.

If someone has dementia (due to whatever underlying cause), it represents an important problem in need of appropriate diagnosis and treatment by a well-trained healthcare provider who specializes in degenerative diseases.

In a nutshell, dementia is a symptom, and AD is the cause of the symptom.

When someone is told they have dementia, it means that they have significant memory problems as well as other cognitive difficulties, and that these problems are severe enough to get in the way of daily living.

Most of the time, dementia is caused by the specific brain disease, AD. However, some uncommon degenerative causes of dementia include vascular dementia (also referred to as multi-infarct dementia), frontotemporal dementia, Lewy Body disease, and chronic traumatic encephalopathy.

Contrary to what some people may think, dementia is not a less severe problem, with AD being a more severe problem. There is not a continuum with dementia on one side and AD at the extreme. Rather, there can be early or mild stages of AD, which then progress to moderate and severe stages of the disease.

One reason for the confusion about dementia and AD is that it is not possible to diagnose AD with 100% accuracy while someone is alive. Rather, AD can only truly be diagnosed after death, upon autopsy when the brain tissue is carefully examined by a specialized doctor referred to as a neuropathologist.

During life, a patient can be diagnosed with "probable AD." This term is used by doctors and researchers to indicate that, based on the person's symptoms, the course of the symptoms, and the results of various tests, it is very likely that the person will show pathological features of AD when the brain tissue is examined following death.

CHAPTER THREE

Types of Dementia

DEMENTIA HAS DIFFERENT types and the classification is mainly based on the whether the intensity of symptoms can be reversed or areas of brain affected.

1. Alzheimer's disease

Alzheimer's disease is the most common type of dementia frequently seen in the age group of 65 years or above. Reports suggest that about 4 million people in the United States are suffering from this disease.

About 360,000 new cases of Alzheimer's disease are reported every year and 50,000 Americans die annually. In the majority of the individuals, the symptoms appear after the age of 60 but the early onset of symptoms is linked to genes.

The disease causes a gradual decline in the cognitive ability of an individual within 7-10 years, and nearly all brain functions associated with memory, movement, language, judgment, behavior and abstract thinking are badly affected. Two chief abnormalities of brain are typically associated with Alzheimer's disease, namely amyloid plaques and neurofibrillary tangles.

Amyloid plaques are unusual clumps of protein (beta amyloid) containing degenerating bits of neurons and other cells that are present in the tissues between the nerve cells. Neurofibrillary tangles are bundles of twisted filaments present within the neurons and are chiefly made up of a protein known as tau.

In healthy neurons, tau protein helps in the functioning of microtubules but in this disease, they twist to form helical filaments that join in the form of tangles, resulting in disintegration of microtubules.

Early symptoms of the disease are identified by memory impairment, subtle changes in personality and judgment inabilities. As the disease progresses, symptoms associated with memory and language become worse and the individual finds difficulty in performing daily activities.

Individuals may often suffer from visuo-spatial problems like difficulty in navigating an unfamiliar route, may become disoriented about time and places, may even suffer from delusions and may become short tempered and hostile. In late stages, the person loses his control over motor functions and may feel difficulty in swallowing, lose bowel and bladder control. They also lose ability to recognize family members.

A person's emotions and behavior get affected in later stages and he may also develop symptoms of aggression, agitation, depression and delusions. A person survives for 8-10 years after the disease diagnosis but some may live for about 20 years or more. Individuals may often die due to aspiration pneumonia as they lose the ability to swallow food.

2. Vascular dementia

Vascular dementia is the second most common cause of dementia after Alzheimer's disease. It is resultant of brain damage by cerebrovascular or cardiovascular problems and accounts for 20% of all types of dementias. Genetic diseases, endocarditis and amyloid angiopathy also play an important role.

It is also known to co-exist with Alzheimer's disease whose incidence increases with advancing age and equally affects both men and women in proportion. Symptoms usually appear suddenly after a stroke.

Patients may have a history of high blood pressure, vascular disease or heart attacks. In some cases, the symptoms recover with time. Vascular dementia is known to affect mid-brain regions to bring changes in the cognitive ability of a person. Individuals may often suffer from depression and incontinence.

Several types of vascular dementia are known to differ from each other on account of their causes and symptoms, for example, multi-infarct dementia (MID) are caused by the presence of numerous small strokes in the brain. This type also includes multiple damaged brain areas and lesions in the white matter, nerves of brain.

As multi-infarct dementia affects only isolated areas of brain, only one or few specific functions of the body are affected. The possibilities of dementia are increased if the left side of brain or hippocampus is damaged.

Another type of dementia is Binswanger's disease, a rare disease where blood vessels of white matter are damaged leading to memory loss, brain lesions, disordered cognition and mood changes.

Patients may often show symptoms of high blood pressure, stroke, blood abnormalities, and disease of large blood vessels of the neck and heart valves.

Other important symptoms include urinary incontinence, difficulty in walking, clumsiness, slowness, lack of facial expression and speech difficulty. The symptoms usually arise after the age of 60 and the treatment includes medications to control high blood pressure and depression.

3. Lewy body dementia (LBD)

Lewy body dementia (LBD) is one of the most common types of progressive dementia, sporadically occurring in individuals with no known familiar history of the disease. The cells in the brain's cortex and substantia nigra die while the remaining cells of the substantia nigra contain abnormal structures known as Lewy bodies that are the hallmark of this disease.

Lewy bodies may also invade the cortex and are made up of a protein (alpha-synuclein) associated with Parkinson's disease and other disorders. Researchers have failed to give satisfactory answers about the accumulation of this protein in the nerve cells.

The symptoms of this form of dementia may overlap with symptoms of Alzheimer's disease in many ways and include memory impairment, confusion and judgment inability.

The typical symptoms include hallucinations, shuffling gait, flexed posture. The individuals may live for 7 years after disease diagnosis. In the present scenario, this form of dementia lacks any cure and the treatments include controlling parkinsonian's and psychiatric symptoms of the disease.

Studies have shown that some neuroleptic drugs like clozapine and olanzapine give positive results against psychiatric symptoms but may cause side effects. The brains of persons suffering from Parkinson's and Alzheimer's disease frequently contain Lewy bodies.

4. Fronto-temporal dementia (FTD)

Fronto-temporal dementia is also known as frontal lobe dementia and is characterized by the degeneration of the nerve cells of the frontal and temporal lobes of brain. This disorder, however, lacks amyloid plaques but neurofibrillary tangles are present that disrupt normal activities of cells resulting in their death.

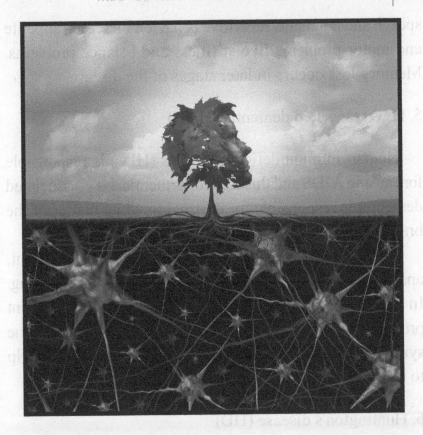

Experts believe that fronto-temporal dementia accounts for about 2-10% of all cases of dementia. The symptoms usually appear between the ages of 40 and 65. In some cases, people have a familiar history of the disease and in such cases, genetic factors strongly influence the disease. People with this disorder may live up to 5-10 years after the diagnosis of the disease.

The frontal and temporal lobes of brain are concerned with judgment and social behavior but in this disorder, as the nerve cells are destroyed, the individual finds it difficult to make decisions as well as maintain social communication. Other possible symptoms include loss of speech and language, repetitive behavior, increased appetite and motor problems like stiffness and balance problems. Memory loss occurs in later stages of the disease.

5. HIV-associated dementia (HAD)

Human immunodeficiency virus (HIV) is responsible for causing AIDS and this form of dementia. HIV-associated dementia is responsible for destroying white matter of the brain.

The typical symptoms include memory impairment, apathy, social withdrawal and difficulty in concentrating. In later stages, individuals may often develop movement problems. No promising drugs are yet available to cure the symptoms but the drugs used for treating AIDS may help to reduce some symptoms.

6. Huntington's disease (HD)

Huntington's disease is a hereditary disorder caused by a wrong gene forming a protein known as huntingtin, and the children of individuals suffering from this disease have a 50% chance of acquiring the gene. Many regions of the brain and spinal cord are destroyed.

The symptoms usually arise in the thirties and forties and a person may live for 15 years after the disease diagnosis. The typical symptoms include mild personality changes like anxiety, irritability, depression, and muscle weakness, arrhythmic movements of body, clumsiness and gait disturbances.

7. Dementia pugilistica

This disorder is also known as chronic traumatic encephalopathy or Boxer's syndrome caused by severe brain injury. Most common symptoms include dementia and Parkinsonism and affected individuals show slurred speech and poor co-ordination. A single brain injury may also cause post-traumatic dementia (PTD) characterized by long term memory problems.

8. Corticobasal degeneration (CBD)

It is a progressive disorder characterized by atrophy of multiple areas of the brain and loss of nerve cells. Brain cells show abnormal accumulation of tau protein, and the disease takes 6-8 years for the development of symptoms that include poor co-ordination and rigidity, similar to those found in Parkinson's disease.

Other symptoms include memory loss, dementia, visuo-spatial problems, apraxia, halting speech and difficulty in swallowing. Death may occur due to pneumonia or other pulmonary infections. There is no effective treatment available for corticobasal degeneration disease but drugs like clonazepam can be used to cure some primary symptoms.

9. Creutzfeldt-Jakob disease (CJD)

This is a rare, degenerative but fatal brain disorder affecting a very small percentage of persons. The symptoms usually arise at the age of 60 and the person dies within a year.

Many researchers believe that this disorder is the result of an abnormal protein known as prion. About 5-10% cases reported in the United States share a genetic basis where this form of dementia is caused by a mutation in the gene for the prion protein.

Patients with Creutzfeldt-Jakob disease suffer from the problems associated with muscle coordination, personality changes, impaired memory, judgment making, thinking disability and impaired vision.

Other possible symptoms include insomnia and depression. In later stages, the persons may also develop myoclonus and may become blind. They finally lose the power to speak and enter coma. Pneumonia and other infections may also be responsible for the death of the individual.

10. Normal Pressure Hydrocephalus (NPH)

Normal pressure hydrocephalus involves an accumulation of cerebrospinal fluid in the brain's cavities. When this fluid does not drain as it should, the associated build-up results in added pressure on the brain, interfering with the brain's ability to function normally.

Individuals with dementia caused by normal pressure hydrocephalus often experience problems with ambulation, balance and bladder control, as well as cognitive impairments involving speech, problem-solving abilities and memory.

11. Wernicke-Korsakoff Syndrome

Wernicke-Korsakoff syndrome is caused by a vitamin B1 (Thiamine)deficiency and often occurs in alcoholics, although it can also result from malnutrition, cancers, abnormally high thyroid hormone levels, long-term dialysis and long-term diuretic therapy (used to treat congestive heart failure).

The symptoms include confusion, permanent gaps in memory, and impaired short-term memory. Hallucinations may also occur. If treated early by supplement, this dementia can be reversed.

12. Mild Cognitive Impairment (MCI)

Dementia can be due to illness, medications and a host of other treatable causes. With mild cognitive impairment, an individual will experience memory loss, and sometimes impaired judgment and speech, but they are usually aware of this decline. These problems usually don't interfere with the normal activities of daily living.

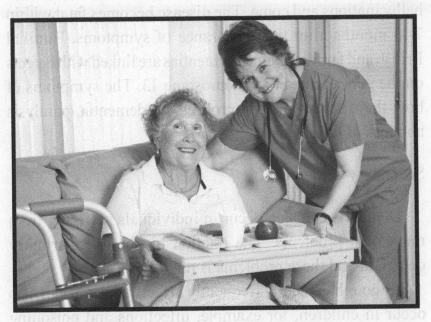

Individuals with mild cognitive impairment may also experience behavioral changes that involve depression, anxiety, aggression and emotional apathy. This is often due to the awareness of and frustration related to his or her condition.

13. Other rare hereditary dementias

They include Gerstmann-Straussler-Scheinker (GSS) disease, fatal familial insomnia, familial British dementia and familial Danish dementia.

Symptoms of Gerstmann-Straussler-Scheinker (GSS) disease include ataxia and progressive dementia occurring at the age of 50-60, and may persist till the death of the individual. Fatal familial insomnia is characterized by damaged thalamus that upsets the sleep of an individual.

Other symptoms include dementia, poor reflexes, hallucinations and coma. The disease becomes fatal within 7-13 months after the appearance of symptoms. Familial British and familial Danish dementias are linked with defects on the gene located on chromosome 13. The symptoms of both the diseases include progressive dementia, paralysis and loss of balance.

Secondary dementias

Dementia can also occur in individuals suffering from movement problems. The relationship between primary dementia and these problems is not clear.

Although dementia frequently affects adults, it can also occur in children, for example, infections and poisoning may lead to dementia in individuals of any age. Some disorders unique to children may also cause dementia.

Niemann-Pick disease is a type of inherited disorder where specific gene mutations affect metabolism of cholesterol, so excessive amounts of cholesterol accumulates in the liver and spleen while excessive lipids accumulate in the brain.

The symptoms include dementia, confusion and problems of learning and memory. The disease is known to affect young school age children but may also affect teenagers.

Batten disease is also a fatal hereditary disorder of the central nervous system occurring in childhood. The symptoms include formation of lipopigments in body tissues and early symptoms include personality and behavior changes, clumsiness or stumbling. As the disease advances, children may experience mental impairment, loss of sight and motor skills, become blind and bedridden.

Lafora body disease is a rare genetic disorder responsible for causing progressive dementia and movement problems. The symptoms arise in the early childhood or late teens and are characterized by the presence of Lafora body's in the brain, skin, muscles and liver, with the death of the child within 2-10 years.

With an understanding of the types of dementia, questions begin to arise about how these diseases are diagnosed. What can a patient expect when trying to determine whether he or she has some form of dementia? What can a caregiver expect?

When you initially meet with your doctor, it is important to be honest with them about the symptoms the patient is experiencing, their duration, frequency and rate of progression. The doctor will then review your current health status, family history and medication history.

This includes evaluating the patient for depression, substance abuse and nutrition, and other conditions that can cause memory loss, including anemia, vitamin deficiency, diabetes, kidney or liver disease, thyroid disease, infections, cardiovascular and pulmonary problems. The patient also undergoes a physical exam and blood tests.

Diagnosing specific diseases causing dementia can be difficult and it may be necessary to ask for a referral to a doctor with expertise in this area. Additional tests that may be used in conjunction with the aforementioned approaches include the Mini Mental State Evaluation (MMSE), the Mini Cog Screen, and Medical Imaging (CT, MRI and PET scans).

The MMSE is an evaluation of the patient's cognitive status. The patient is required to identify the time, date and place where the test is taking place, be able to count backwards, identify objects previously known to him or her, be able to repeat common phrases, perform basic skills involving math, language use and comprehension, and demonstrate basic motor skills.

The Mini Cog Screen takes only a few minutes to administer, and is used as an initial screening for dementia. The patient is required to identify three objects in the office, then draw the face of a clock in its entirety from memory, and finally, recall the three items identified earlier.

Finally, medical imaging helps doctors see images of the patient's brain to determine whether there are any growths, abnormalities or general shrinkage which occurs in Alzheimer's disease. These medical imaging tests can help improve the accuracy of a dementia diagnosis to 90%.

Once a diagnosis has been made, doctors can help patients to look at various treatment options and can often provide information for caregivers and families about support groups and organizations that can provide them with information about their specific diagnosis.

It is recommended that patients and their families try to learn as much as they can about the disease and how it is expected to progress.

Organizations like Alzheimer's Society or the Parkinsons Society can provide valuable information about the disease, its progression, and tips on how to slow the progression of the disease and deal with symptoms. These organizations also provide support groups to both the patient and their caregivers to help deal with the blow of a dementia diagnosis.

As mentioned earlier, early detection is often key in being able to reverse or slow the progression of many of these diseases. Having a basic understanding of the many dementias that may occur and how they are diagnosed will be beneficial to physicians and families alike.

If you find that you simply do not know where to begin or how to handle this change in status and what it means for your future, a Geriatric Care Manager can assist you in making plans for the future.

CHAPTER FOUR
Causes and Diagnosis of Dementia

THE EARLY WARNING SIGNS

ALZHEIMER'S DISEASE IS generally associated with elderly people as it often begins over the age of 65, and the greater the age, the greater the risk, however, there is also an early form of Alzheimer's disease that is relatively rare but which progresses more rapidly.

Both men and women can develop Alzheimer's but women seem to be slightly more at risk than men. Other risk factors include medical conditions affecting the heart and arteries, environmental factors such as smoking, and diet.

There isn't a definitive cause, neither is there an established genetic link, although research is currently being done in this area as some families do seem to show a genetic tendency, particularly if two direct relatives have the disease.

Other environmental causes that have been suggested in the past include exposure to magnetic fields, or to aluminium, but these have never been scientifically validated.

What are the early signs and symptoms?

The most common early symptom reported is memory lapses. Although some memory loss is perfectly normal as we age, in people with Alzheimer's disease, there is a much faster decline as well as other cognitive problems that become increasingly evident.

It is usually the sufferer's family and friends that will first notice that someone isn't behaving in the way that they used to.

For example, short term memory lapses become more common and the individual finds it difficult to concentrate on tasks that they once found easy. Personality changes may become evident as well as problems with communication.

Early signs and symptoms of Alzheimer's disease can include any or all of the following:

- Confusion
- Apathy
- Avoiding social contact

- Irritability and anxiousness
- Forgetting names and places on a regular basis
- Repeating oneself often in a short space of time
- An inability to get organised, plan and think coherently
- Difficulty with daily routine tasks and making decisions
- Difficulty with arithmetic, reading, writing and other cognitive tasks
- May become disorientated in familiar places
- Indulging in strange behaviour

It is important to note that these symptoms do not necessarily indicate that someone is in the early stages of Alzheimer's disease as these same symptoms can occur as a result of other completely unconnected factors.

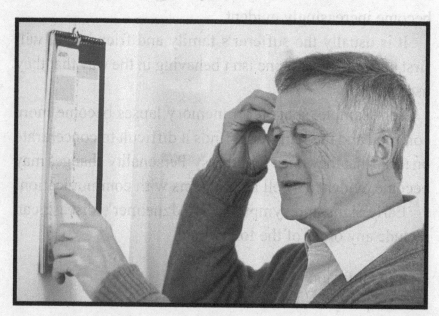

In the early stages, an individual may be able to compensate quite well for these problems and will continue to live and work independently for some time. However, the nature of Alzheimer's is that the symptoms will always get progressively worse, and severe dementia is inevitable.

What is the prognosis?

There is no cure for Alzheimer's disease so treatment is of a palliative nature. As the disease progresses, an individual's ability to function independently will decline until eventually, they lose control of their mental faculties and all bodily functions.

If the disease is diagnosed early, then there is some evidence that with a good diet and the right kind of support and care, it may be possible to delay the progression of the disease; however, this is not conclusive.

One of the most devastating aspects of this disease is the effect it can have on family and friends who are forced to watch their loved one deteriorate to the point that they no longer recognise them. Indeed, there is a higher rate of depression amongst carers of people with Alzheimer's disease than those with Alzheimer's themselves.

Many people with Alzheimer's stay at home, particularly in the early stages, and are cared for by family. There is a great deal that can be done on a practical basis to ensure that the individual suffering from Alzheimer's remains as independent as possible for as long as possible, as well as help and support available for those who care for them.

There are a number of organisations that have been set up with the primary aim of doing just that. You can find out more information about what is available in your area by speaking to your doctor or other health care professional.

Early onset Alzheimer's can often start a lot earlier than many people think. Most of us may think that the Alzheimer's disease mainly affects older people, mainly in their sixties and seventies, when in fact it does affect a lot of younger people as well. This disease has been known to affect people in their early forties.

Most people who get diagnosed with early onset Alzheimer's have developed the disease through their family genes. This means that there is a family history of Alzheimer's disease which, in turn, means that there is a high chance that this disease will be passed on to your siblings as well.

Being diagnosed with Alzheimer's disease can be devastating for any person to come to terms with. What is even worse for some people is that they still have a young family to raise themselves.

Some of these people who have been diagnosed with this awful disease may also be single parents. This makes it even harder for them to cope.

They will not only have to come to terms with all this, but in all likelihood, they will have to give up work as well, meaning that there will be less money coming into the household.

What you will need to do is make sure that you get a lot of help, if possible from family and friends or from an Alzheimer's care giving team. You will also want to get some advice on any benefits you will be able to receive once you have to stop working.

The signs and symptoms of early onset Alzheimer's are similar to the symptoms of late onset Alzheimer's. The symptoms include memory loss, confusion, personality changes, misplacing things, problems with language and it will get to the stage where simple tasks will become too difficult for you to do.

As with late onset Alzheimer's disease, there is no cure for early onset Alzheimer's. There is medication to help slow down the progression of this terrible disease. These drugs are called cholinesterase inhibitors and what they do is to break down the acetylcholine in the brain. This is a substance that occurs naturally in the brain. A person with Alzheimer's disease has a reduced amount of acetylcholine in the brain, and this is why with the loss of this chemical, it starts to interfere with your memory function.

You need to remember that you are not the only one to be diagnosed with early onset Alzheimer's. You'll need to stay positive and concentrate on the things you can do, rather than the things you can't do.

Start to write things down as soon as you think of them. Make sure you keep up your social life. Take all the help you can get. Don't be afraid to ask professional people about your family and your finances. These people are there to help you.

The onset of the disease is gradual but the symptoms become more penetrating as the disease advances. Problems associated with short-term memory normally arise in the earlier phase of the disease.

Mild personality changes also occur in the preliminary phase of the disorder. With the advancement of the disease, the patient develops symptoms of difficulty in abstract thinking and other intellectual impairments.

The patient also finds it difficult to carry out the office work. Behavioral changes also take place. In later cases, the person becomes confused and disoriented in relation to month, time, people and places. The person is also at the jeopardy of getting infected with pneumonia and the condition becomes worse before the death of the patient.

CAUSES

Dementia is the result of death of nerve cells or loss of communication between neurons. The human brain is a very complex machine and a number of factors can alter its proper functioning. Although researchers have found the factors responsible for causing dementia, more precise study is still required.

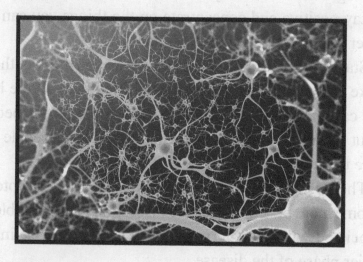

Different types of dementias, for example, Alzheimer's disease, Parkinson's dementia, Pick's disease are identified by the presence of abnormal inclusions in the brain developing symptoms of dementia. Genes also play a very important role in the development of some types of dementias where lifestyle factors and environmental influences are important.

Researchers have identified many genes that increase the susceptibility of an individual to Alzheimer's disease, but among them, the mutation in three genes that control the production of proteins like amyloid precursor protein (APP), presenilin 1 and presenilin 2 is important. Variation in a gene known as apolipoprotein E is responsible for causing late symptoms of Alzheimer's disease.

Studies have also indicated that mutations in another gene, CYP46, increase the risk of late onset of Alzheimer's disease. The gene is responsible for the production of a protein responsible for the brain cholesterol metabolism.

Scientists are working to find out how beta amyloid influences the development of Alzheimer's disease. Vascular dementia may arise due to cerebrovascular disease or any condition that prevents normal blood supply to the brain. When the blood supply to brain cells is insufficient, the cells suffer from oxygen deficiency and finally die.

Diagnosis

Doctors employ a number of strategies while dealing with the individuals suffering from dementia and it is always beneficial to rule out all the conditions that can be easily treated by medications. Disease diagnosis can be done by the following methods:

1. Patient' history

While starting the diagnosis, a doctor may ask about the family background of the patient by asking questions like how and when the symptoms developed as well as what is the overall medical condition of the patient?

The doctor may also try to evaluate the mental state of the patient. Questions can be asked to the family members to learn the family history in order to ensure whether or not the disease has been present in the family earlier.

2. Physical examination

Physical examination of the patient may help to identify the signs or other disorders that can contribute to dementia. It can also identify the presence of heart or kidney disease that may overlap with dementia.

3. Neurological evaluation

Neurological examinations can be performed by doctors to check balance, sensory function, reflexes or other symptoms to see whether or not they can be recovered by drugs.

4. Cognitive and neuropsychological tests

Doctors perform tests to check the memory, language skills, maths skills and other tests in order to find out the mental alertness of the patient.

They can often use a test known as Mini-Mental State Examination (MMSE) which analyses the orientation, memory and attention as well as language commands. Doctors also use other tests with variable scales in order to judge the mental state of the patient.

5. Brain scans

Doctors may use brain scans in order to find out strokes or tumors that can cause symptoms of dementia. Degeneration of the brain's cortex is very common in many types of dementias and brain scans can easily detect it.

The most commonly used brain scans are the computerized tomography (CT) and magnetic resonance imaging (MRI). Doctors frequently use the CT brain scans which use X-rays and can detect changes in brain structures.

MRI scans use magnetic fields and radio waves to detect hydrogen atoms present in body tissues. Medical experts can also use electroencephalogram (EEGs) in case of suspicious individuals.

EEGs record the electrical activity as well as abnormalities in brain structures. Several types of brain scans are available that help the medical experts to keep a check over the brain's activity.

The functional brain scans include MRI (fMRI), single photon-emission computed tomography (SPECT), positron emission tomography (PET) and magnetoencephalography (MEG). fMRI uses radio waves and a strong magnetic field that keeps a regular check on the activities going inside the active parts of the brain.

SPECT increases brain activity by showing the distribution of blood in the brain. PET detects changes in glucose and oxygen metabolism and blood flow, revealing abnormalities in brain function. MEG shows electromagnetic fields caused by neurons of the brain.

6. Laboratory tests

Doctors may use a variety of laboratory tests in order to find out whether or not the individual is suffering from dementia. The list of tests includes total blood count, blood glucose test, urinalysis, drug and alcohol tests, cerebrospinal fluid test, and thyroid gland analysis.

7. Psychiatric evaluation

A psychiatric evaluation is done to check whether the symptoms are due to dementia or if there are some other factors coupled with it.

8. Presymptomatic testing

Testing the individuals before the symptoms appear and develop into dementia is not possible in many cases.

Risk factors for dementia

Researchers have identified many factors that can be held responsible for developing one or other types of dementia. Some of these factors are modifiable while others are not. These factors include:

1. Age

The symptoms of Alzheimer's disease, vascular dementia and other types of dementia generally appear with advancing age.

2. Genetics or family history

Scientists have found a number of genes responsible for causing Alzheimer's disease but persons with a family history of the disease are at an elevated risk of developing the disease.

3. Smoking and alcohol consumption

Smoking and use of alcohol also increases the risk of mental declination and dementia. Individuals who smoke regularly are at an elevated risk of suffering from atherosclerosis and other vascular diseases that can be coupled with dementia.

4. Atherosclerosis

High levels of low-density lipoproteins (LDL), also known as the bad cholesterol, increase the risk of vascular diseases that can be linked with increased risk of Alzheimer's disease.

5. Plasma homocysteine

Researchers have indicated that higher levels of blood homocysteine increase the risk of vascular dementia.

6. Diabetes

Diabetes is also a very common factor associated with many types of dementias as it also increases the risk of atherosclerosis and stroke that ultimately cause vascular dementia.

7. Mild cognitive impairment

People with mild cognitive impairment are at an increased risk of developing dementia, especially if they are above the age of 65 or more.

8. Down syndrome

Studies have shown that individuals suffering from Down syndrome develop amyloid plaques and neurofibrillary tangles in their middle age but not all the individuals develop symptoms of dementia.

Advantages of seeking an early diagnosis

The early symptoms of dementia are very similar to what most people consider a normal part of "aging."

These include symptoms like memory loss, confusion, disorientation, inability to do normal activities, withdrawal, agitation, and frustration. Many patients who face such problems do not consult a doctor, thinking, "This must be normal at my age. I'll look foolish if I go to a doctor with these problems."

On the other hand, when people who know about dementia, experience such symptoms, they suspect (or fear) that they have dementia.

However, they hesitate to consult a doctor because of the stigma of being diagnosed with dementia.

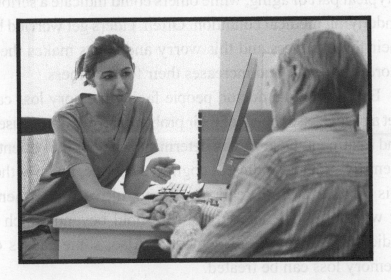

In some cultures, people may associate "dementia" with strange behavior, helplessness, and negativity, and they don't want to be labeled as dementia patients.

In other cultures, where dementia awareness is poor, there is a stigma about a dementia diagnosis because people associate dementia with insanity. People also hesitate to get a diagnosis because they have heard that dementia is incurable, so they see no point in "wasting" time and money by going to a doctor.

There are, however, several advantages of consulting a doctor for investigations and diagnosis as soon as the symptoms are noticed.

These advantages are described below.

Not all memory loss is dementia

There are many types of memory loss. Also, everyone forgets things once in a while. Some memory problems are a typical part of aging, while others could indicate a serious underlying medical condition. Often, elders get worried by their forgetfulness and this worry and stress makes them more inattentive and increases their forgetfulness.

By talking to a doctor, people facing memory loss can get a proper assessment of their problem, its possible causes, and treatment. Doctors can determine whether the patient's memory problem indicates cognitive decline, and whether this decline is mild (called mild cognitive impairment) or whether it has crossed the threshold beyond which it indicates a diagnosis of dementia. Also, some causes of memory loss can be treated.

Sometimes, depression is mistaken for dementia

Depression can reduce the ability to pay attention and can cause memory problems. Lay persons cannot distinguish whether their memory loss and confusion is caused by dementia or by depression. Depression responds well to treatment, and the symptoms can be reversed. Getting a timely diagnosis is therefore useful.

Dementia symptoms are also caused by treatable problems like deficiency of Vitamin B12, hypothyroidism, etc.

Many people think dementia symptoms are caused solely by incurable medical problems (like Alzheimer's). In reality, there are over seventy causes of dementia symptoms. Some of them, like deficiency of Vitamin B12 or hypothyroidism, can be treated, and such treatment will reverse the symptoms of dementia.

A proper diagnosis detects reversible causes which can then be corrected. If a patient does not go to a doctor, he/she continues to suffer unnecessarily.

Knowing that we have mild cognitive impairment affects our life choices

Persons with mild cognitive impairment (MCI) may or may not go on to develop dementia, but the probability of their developing dementia is higher than that of persons without MCI.

If a doctor, on checking a patient, concludes that the patient has MCI, this impacts the decisions the patient may take. For example, though there is no known way to prevent dementia, research suggests that healthy lifestyle choices reduce the risk.

The patient may therefore decide to be more alert about diet, exercise, and other life choices. For example, a person may start an exercise program, become socially active, and quit smoking.

Knowing that he/she has MCI may also affect decisions the person takes about their future.

Early diagnosis means treatment can begin earlier, and years of suffering may be reduced.

As of now, dementias like Alzheimer's Disease cannot be reversed, but there are some medications that aim to improve the patient's quality of life by reducing the symptoms.

While these medications do not work for everyone, a patient who gets an early diagnosis can try out the medication earlier and may experience some relief from the symptoms, and thus lead a better life.

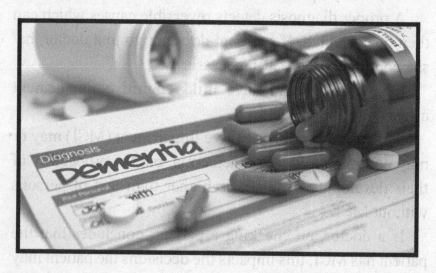

An early diagnosis allows more time for the patient to plan for dementia.

In an early-stage diagnosis, the patient is still mentally alert enough to understand the disease and its possible impacts. Though it may take time to accept the diagnosis, the patient has the mental ability to understand the impact of dementia and start preparing for the years ahead.

An early-stage diagnosis allows patients to discuss their wishes with relatives, arrange their finances, wrap up projects, and generally plan for their future. Patients are also able to talk to friends and relatives, explain the situation, and seek support.

Having the knowledge that their problems are caused by an organic brain disorder reduces their bewilderment and worry, and allows them to focus on what they still can do and orient their lives to make the most of what they have. They can seek counseling and learn more about their condition.

In case of a mid-stage/ late-stage diagnosis, the patient is likely to find the diagnosis more overwhelming, and cannot believe or understand it, let alone plan for the future.

An early diagnosis gives family and friends more time to plan care

A person with dementia needs care, and this care increases as the dementia worsens. Family caregivers need to adjust their lives accordingly; adjustments could include changing jobs, relocating, arranging finances, discussing division of work and responsibilities amongst family members, and so on.

Family members also get more time to understand dementia and pick up the necessary care giving skills, join support groups, get counseling, and so on. The earlier the diagnosis, the smoother it is to support the person with dementia.

Late diagnosis means more suffering for the patient and family

A late diagnosis means that for many years, the person with dementia has been coping with the confusion and reduced ability without knowing why the problems are occurring. This is stressful and unnerving, and the stress worsens the symptoms. If the problem is treatable, all this suffering could have been avoided.

A late diagnosis also means that the family, friends, and colleagues who have been interacting with the patients have been treating the patient as someone with normal memory and abilities.

They have not been making allowances for the memory loss, reduced ability, and confusion. Because of this, they have been (without intending to) stressing the patients by expecting them to understand and remember things, and to handle complex decisions.

Family members may have shown impatience when the patient forgot things, acted clumsily, or behaved in strange ways. The patient's frustration, rage, or withdrawal may upset family members who don't understand that this is caused by dementia.

Because the family members do not know about the dementia, they do not take steps to prevent the patient from self-harm or from harming others. For example, the patient may continue to drive, even after it is not advisable, or may wander, or leave equipment and kitchen gadgets unattended, or not be watchful enough if asked to babysit an infant.

A person who experiences symptoms of memory loss or functioning that hampers normal life should consult a medical professional to determine the cause and severity.

Also, alert family members should ensure that a check-up is done. Perhaps the symptoms are caused by a problem that can be treated. Perhaps the symptoms are not dementia.

And even if the symptoms are caused by an irreversible dementia, an early diagnosis allows starting treatment to alleviate the symptoms, and also allows the patient and the family more time to plan for the future.

BLOOD TEST THAT DETECTS EARLY ALZHEIMER'S DISEASE

What makes Alzheimer's disease such a terrifying prospect is the inevitability of it all. We have no vaccines or preventive measures, so you either get Alzheimer's or you don't. Once you have it, there's little hope of recovery, because we have no treatment or cure.

But what if we could detect the disease years before its symptoms start to appear, to not only give patients the chance to slow the progression, but also give researchers better insight into how it develops?

A 'proof of concept' trial of a new blood test has just been completed, and the team behind it has reported "unparalleled accuracy" in detecting the early stages of Alzheimer's.

"It is now generally believed that Alzheimer's-related changes begin in the brain at least a decade before the emergence of telltale symptoms," says one of the team,

Robert Nagele from the Rowan University School of Osteopathic Medicine and Durin Technologies, Inc.

"To the best of our knowledge, this is the first blood test using autoantibody biomarkers that can accurately detect Alzheimer's at an early point in the course of the disease when treatments are more likely to be beneficial - that is, before too much brain devastation has occurred."

The test is designed to detect an early stage of Alzheimer's disease called mild cognitive impairment (MCI), and distinguish it from similar cases of mental decline that are caused by other factors such as vascular issues, chronic depression, alcohol abuse, and the side effects of certain drugs.

For the trial, Nagele and his team took blood samples from 236 participants, including 50 who had been diagnosed with MCI, 50 with mild-moderate Alzheimer's disease, 50 healthy controls, and the remainder had been diagnosed with mild-moderate Parkinson's disease, early-stage Parkinson's, multiple sclerosis, or breast cancer.

The MCI patients had been diagnosed based on having low levels of amyloid-beta 42 peptide in their cerebrospinal fluid, which has been identified as a predictor of rapid Alzheimer's progression.

To analyse the blood, the test uses a number of human protein microarrays - catalogues of 9,486 unique human proteins - to send out proteins to attract autoantibodies in the blood that could be linked to the disease.

Autoantibodies are a particular type of antibody produced by the immune system to target certain proteins in the body. This can sometimes go horribly wrong, and end up as an autoimmune disease, but the way they respond to different types of diseases has made them a very promising new candidate for detection and diagnosis.

The researchers identified the 50 best autoantibody biomarkers for MCI and the other diseases diagnosed in their participants, and when they used these to analyse the blood samples, they found them to be 100 percent accurate in the overall accuracy, sensitivity and specificity rate in detecting the blood samples from participants with MCI.

Using this biomarker method, the test was also successful in detecting mild-moderate Alzheimer's (98.7 percent), early-stage Parkinson's disease (98.0 percent), multiple sclerosis (100 percent) and breast cancer (100 percent).

The team says that while these results are exciting, they need to test the method on a much larger and more diverse sample, to see if that 100 percent average wavers with additional data.

While at this stage, knowing that you have Alzheimer's earlier rather than later, won't prevent it from developing altogether, it could give patients the opportunity to sign up for clinical trials for new drugs and treatments, plan out future medical care, and even explore ways to help delay its progression, the team reports in the journal Alzheimer's & Dementia.

With the disease affecting approximately 5.3 million people in the US, including almost half of the population at 85 years and older, we need tests like this. And who knows? Maybe if we get to know Alzheimer's better in its early stages, we might just be able to figure out how it begins, and how to prevent it.

Other conditions causing dementia

Doctors have found many conditions that can cause dementia and some symptoms can be reversed with proper treatment. For example, medications can sometimes cause symptoms of dementia.

They can be caused either by a single drug or by the activity of multiple drug interactions. Thyroid problems can also cause depression and dementia. Hypoglycemia also causes confusion and personality changes.

Too high or too low sodium and calcium levels can also result in mental problems. Some individuals are unable to absorb vitamin B12 so they suffer from pernicious anemia resulting in personality changes, irritability or depression. Thiamine deficiency resulting from chronic alcoholism can also cause mental impairment.

Severe deficiency of vitamin B6 causes pellagra resulting in dementia. Dehydration can also cause mental illness. Many infections cause neurological illness that develop symptoms of dementia, for example, meningitis and encephalitis cause severe mental impairment, judgment problems or memory loss. Untreated syphilis also causes dementia.

A rare disease known as Lyme disease also causes dementia. Individuals suffering from leukemia and AIDS develop an infection known as progressive multifocal leukoencephalopathy (PML) that causes mental illness. Subdural hematomas also cause symptoms of dementia and other mental problems.

Exposure to lead, other heavy metals or other toxic elements also cause dementia. The symptoms may or may not be reversed as they depend upon the total area of brain damaged. Individuals who consume alcohol or other recreational drugs also show symptoms of dementia; the responses are short lasting and the condition is known as substance-induced persisting dementia.

Even individuals with brain tumors may also suffer from dementia as their brains are damaged. The symptoms include personality changes, speech and language problems and memory loss. Anoxia is caused by heart attacks, heart surgery, asthma, high altitude exposure or smoke also develops symptoms of dementia.

CHAPTER FIVE

Stages of Alzheimer's Disease

ALZHEIMER'S DISEASE is an illness that sneaks in and attacks a victim without warning. Once it establishes its foundation, it slowly robs the victim of time, energy, function, and perhaps the most precious thing of all, memories.

It seems the old adage, "No one can take this from you," doesn't hold true anymore. Alzheimer's disease starts with mild symptoms, and slowly progresses and interferes with everyday functioning and even impairs simple judgment and movement.

The seven stages of Alzheimer's disease have been documented in correspondence directly with underlying nerve cell degeneration. The damage to nerve cells begins to affect the victim with memory and learning. Nerve cell damage gradually affects every day thinking, judgment, and behavior.

Alzheimer's disease is unique in that it does not manifest itself with the same symptoms in every victim. Many times, a person diagnosed with Alzheimer's disease will not show signs of their illness for years after diagnosis.

Survival of victims once diagnosed, can be anywhere from three to twenty years. Medical science has established a Global Deterioration Scale, which corresponds directly with underlying nerve cell damage that takes place with Alzheimer's disease.

Global Deterioration Scale

Stage One

No signs of impairment. During this stage, individuals will typically show no signs of memory or impairment of judgement. They present no evidence of Alzheimer's disease to the health care professional.

Stage Two

Mild cognitive impairment. Individuals in this stage will typically present with very mild symptoms of Alzheimer's disease. Symptoms during this stage will typically manifest themselves with short memory lapses, such as forgetting everyday items such as car keys, and television remotes. It is difficult to detect symptoms at this stage for the health care professional.

Stage Three

This is the stage where individuals begin to show consistent signs of Alzheimer's disease to family, and may be easily detected by the health care professional. Detecting Alzheimer's disease during this stage will usually be noticed by close family members, or the closest of friends of the individual.

Common symptoms during this stage may be forgetting simple short passages of reading material, misplacing common everyday items, decrease in ability to organize and plan events, difficulty in remembering names of new people, and not finding the right words during discussions with other people.

Stage Four

Moderate cognitive deficits. This is also called mild or early stage Alzheimer's disease. During this stage, a health care professional will detect deficiencies and knowledge of recent current events, difficulty to perform easy mental arithmetic, decreased ability to plan events such as dinner, decreased memory of personal history, and social withdrawal from close friends.

Stage Five

Moderate to severe cognitive decline. This is also called moderate or main stage Alzheimer's disease. Memory deficits are much more severe during this stage. The health care provider can usually detect Alzheimer's disease very easily during this stage.

Common symptoms include the inability to recall important details in personal life such as address or phone number, counting backwards, difficulty in choosing clothing for the season or current weather conditions, forgetting where common items are placed such as car keys, television remotes, and other items used commonly.

Stage Six

Severe cognitive deficits. This is also called moderate to severe or main stage Alzheimer's disease. Memory difficulties are worse than stage five. Individuals' personalities are affected and they may begin to withdraw or manifest severe personality changes or disorders.

The health care professional will commonly detect an inability to recall current events and events that took place in the last three months, inability to recall personal history, inability to recognize close family members consistently, inability to dress for current weather conditions, and difficulty or inability to perform personal hygiene tasks. The individual may also show signs of wandering, or hallucinating intermittently.

Stage Seven

Very severe cognitive deficits. This is also called severe or late stage Alzheimer's disease. This is the final stage of Alzheimer's disease and manifests itself in individuals with an inability to respond properly to their environment, inability to speak properly, inability to complete coordinated muscle movements.

The health care provider will also commonly detect an individual's inability to speak clearly, recall current events, recognize close family members consistently, inability or severe difficulty with walking or transferring, and inability to swallow.

The Global Deterioration Scale is a system developed by medical professionals and helps to categorize each individual in a certain stage of this unique disease. Proper diagnosis and determination of which stage an individual may be in is critical to the proper care of the individual.

The improvement and rehabilitation of each individual is dependent upon proper diagnosis and placement within the proper stage. Some individuals have been documented to show some level of improvement with proper intervention.

CHAPTER SIX
Importance of Clinical Evaluation

NO SPECIFIC BLOOD test and imaging technique can predict whether a person is suffering from Alzheimer's disease. For the diagnosis of this disorder, a person must fulfill the criteria that forms the baseline for dementia.

A number of factors can be considered responsible for the development of dementia. Neurological disorders, namely Parkinson's disease, brain tumors, blood clots, cerebrovascular disease and strokes can be sometimes associated with dementia. Chronic syphilis, chronic HIV can also sometimes develop the symptoms of dementia.

Many medications, namely those used for the control of bladder urgency and incontinence, can also cause cognitive impairment. Psychiatric and neurological medications are also responsible for cognitive impairment. If the medical expert finds these medication problems in the patient, he strongly recommends halting the usage of these drugs.

Older individuals that usually suffer from depression can also develop the problems associated with memory and concentration loss and such a condition can be specified as pseudodementia. Excessive use of alcohol and illegal drugs can be sometimes responsible for the symptoms of dementia.

Thyroid dysfunction, thiamine deficiency and steroid disorders can also lead to cognitive impairment. Blood clots outside the brain region can also cause symptoms of dementia. Carbon monoxide poisoning leads to encephalopathy that develops symptoms of dementia. Sometimes, heavy metal poisoning is also considered responsible for dementia.

Since a number of disorders are often confused with Alzheimer's disease, a comprehensive clinical evaluation is very important for the accurate diagnosis of the disease. Three procedures are generally followed while diagnosing the disorder and these are a complete medical workup, neurological examination and psychiatric evaluation.

These evaluations usually continue for at least an hour. In the United States healthcare system, a combined help of neurologists, psychiatrics and geriatrics is taken. Even a single physician can also perform the evaluation well. The American Academy of Neurology has given some guidelines that include brain imaging while working with the patients of dementia.

These imaging techniques comprise a non-contrast CT scan or MRI scan. SPECT, fMRI, PET can also be of help but are not used. In areas outside the United States, brain imaging is considered an important factor in diagnosing Alzheimer's disease. The search for an efficient blood test for the perfect diagnosis of Alzheimer's disease is still going on.

Prognosis

Alzheimer's disease is customarily a progressive disorder that reaches its peak within the interval of 8-15 years. The patients generally do not die with the disorder alone but they also suffer from a number of others problems like difficulty in swallowing, walking and patients are at an elevated risk of getting infected with pneumonia.

In the later courses of the disease, strong family assistance is required. A patient of Alzheimer's disease is, however, unable to solve numerical problems but can be interested in reading a magazine.

Playing the piano may be too difficult for the patient as he can make many mistakes but the ability to sing and listen to music remains unaffected. Playing chess may be too difficult for the patient but he or she may feel pleasure in playing tennis.

CHAPTER SEVEN

Prevention of Alzheimer's Disease

ALZHEIMER'S DISEASE is one of the most dreaded nervous system diseases, affecting many people as they advance in age. The most common cause of dementia, Alzheimer's disease increases in prevalence in the elderly, although it can occasionally prevent earlier in life.

This degenerative disease leads to the slow deterioration of nervous system function, particularly affecting cognition, leading to memory loss, confusion, mood swings, and deterioration of other higher brain function. Currently, there is no cure and Alzheimer's is a chronic and terminal disease, generally progressing to death after many years.

While research has elucidated many of the changes that occur in the brain in patients with Alzheimer's, the initiating cause is poorly understood.

Abnormal plaques and "tangles" are found in the brains of patients, but the factors or underlying etiology which leads to their formation is a hotly debated topic. The cause is probably multifactorial with many factors which predispose to the disease in concert.

So what can we do? Is there any way to prevent the disease before it is too late? Unfortunately, there have been no studies that have shown that any one measure is strongly effective in preventing Alzheimer's disease.

Some studies have suggested some links which may predict which people are at the highest risk for developing the disease. Some of these risks cannot be modified, such as genetic factors or advancing age. However, others, such as diet, are modifiable and can potentially decrease the risk of the disease.

What are the best ways to reduce the risk of Alzheimer's?

The thought of developing Alzheimer's disease as you get older can be a frightening prospect, especially if you've witnessed a loved one affected by the disease. Researchers across the world are racing towards a cure, but as prevalence rates climb, their focus has broadened from treatment to prevention strategies.

What they've discovered is that it may be possible to prevent or delay the symptoms of Alzheimer's disease and other dementias through a combination of healthy habits.

By identifying and controlling your personal risk factors, you can maximize your chances of lifelong brain health and take effective steps to preserve your cognitive abilities.

The 6 pillars for reducing your risk

6 Pillars of Brain Health

Alzheimer's is a complex disease with multiple risk factors. Some, like your age and genetics, are outside your control. However, there are six pillars for a brain-healthy lifestyle that are within your control.

The more you strengthen each of the six pillars in your daily life, the longer—and stronger—your brain will stay working.

1: Regular exercise

According to the Alzheimer's Research & Prevention Foundation, regular physical exercise can reduce your risk of developing Alzheimer's disease by up to 50 percent.

What's more, exercise can also slow further deterioration in those who have already started to develop cognitive problems. Exercise protects against Alzheimer's by stimulating the brain's ability to maintain old connections as well as make new ones.

Aim for at least 150 minutes of moderate intensity exercise each week. The ideal plan involves a combination of cardio exercise and strength training. Good activities for beginners include walking and swimming.

Build muscle to pump up your brain. Moderate levels of weight and resistance training not only increase muscle mass, they help you maintain brain health. For those over 65, adding 2-3 strength sessions to your weekly routine may cut your risk of Alzheimer's in half.

Include balance and coordination exercises. Head injuries from falls are an increasing risk as you age, which in turn increase your risk for Alzheimer's disease and dementia. Balance and coordination exercises can help you stay agile and avoid spills. Try yoga, Tai Chi, or exercises using balance balls.

Tips for starting and sticking with an exercise plan

Protect your head

Head trauma at any point in life may increase your risk of Alzheimer's disease. This includes repeated hits in sports activities such as football, soccer, and boxing, or one-time injuries from a bicycle, skating, or motorcycle accident. Protect your brain by wearing properly fitting sports helmets and trip-proofing your environment as you exercise. Avoid activities that compete for your attention— like talking on your cell while walking or cycling.

If you've been inactive for a while, starting an exercise program can be intimidating. But remember: a little exercise is better than none. In fact, adding just modest amounts of physical activity to your weekly routine can have a profound effect on your health.

Choose activities you enjoy and start small—a 10-minute walk a few times a day, for example—and allow yourself to gradually build up your momentum and self-confidence. It takes about 28 days for a new routine to become habit, so do your best to stick with it for a month and soon your exercise routine will feel natural, even something you'll miss if you skip a session.

2: Social engagement

Human beings are highly social creatures. We don't thrive in isolation, and neither do our brains. Staying socially engaged may even protect against Alzheimer's disease and dementia in later life, so make developing and maintaining a strong network of friends a priority.

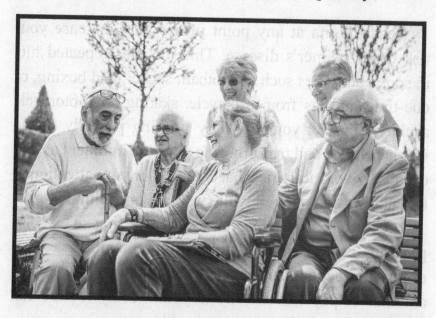

You don't need to be a social butterfly or the life of the party, but you do need to regularly connect face-to-face with someone who cares about you and makes you feel heard. While many of us become more isolated as we get older, it's never too late to meet others and develop new friendships:

- Volunteer
- Join a club or social group
- Visit your local community center or senior center
- Take group classes (such as at the gym or a community college)
- Reach out over the phone or email
- Connect to others via social networks such as Facebook
- Get to know your neighbors
- Make a weekly date with friends
- Get out (go to the movies, the park, museums, and other public places)

3: Healthy diet

In Alzheimer's disease, inflammation and insulin resistance injure neurons and inhibit communication between brain cells. Alzheimer's is sometimes described as "diabetes of the brain," and a growing body of research suggests a strong link between metabolic disorders and the signal processing systems. By adjusting your eating habits, however, you can help reduce inflammation and protect your brain.

Healthy eating tips

Cut down on sugar. Sugary foods and refined carbs such as white flour, white rice, and pasta can lead to dramatic spikes in blood sugar which inflame your brain. Watch out for hidden sugar in all kinds of packaged foods from cereals and bread to pasta sauce and low or no-fat products.

Enjoy a Mediterranean diet. Several epidemiological studies show that eating a Mediterranean diet dramatically reduces the risk of cognitive imapairment and Alzheimer's disease. That means plenty of vegetables, beans, whole grains, fish and olive oil—and limited processed food.

Avoid trans-fats. These fats can cause inflammation and produce free radicals—both of which are hard on the brain. Reduce your consumption by avoiding fast food, fried and packaged foods, and anything that contains "partially hydrogenated oils," even if it claims to be trans-fat-free.

Get plenty of omega-3 fats. Evidence suggests that the DHA found in these healthy fats may help prevent Alzheimer's disease and dementia by reducing beta-amyloid plaques. Food sources include cold-water fish such as salmon, tuna, trout, mackerel, seaweed, and sardines. You can also supplement with fish oil.

Stock up on fruit and vegetables. When it comes to fruits and vegetables, the more the better. Eat up across the color spectrum to maximize protective antioxidants and vitamins, including green leafy vegetables, berries, and cruciferous vegetables such as broccoli.

Enjoy daily cups of tea. Regular consumption of great tea may enhance memory and mental alertness and slow brain aging. White and oolong teas are also particularly brain healthy. Drinking 2-4 cups daily has proven benefits, and although not as powerful as tea, coffee also confers brain benefits.

Cook at home often. By cooking at home, you can ensure that you're eating fresh, wholesome meals that are high in brain-healthy nutrients and low in sugar, salt, unhealthy fat, and additives.

Supplements that may help prevent dementia

Folic acid, vitamin B12, vitamin D, magnesium, and fish oil may help to preserve brain health. Studies of vitamin E, ginkgo biloba, coenzyme Q10, and turmeric have yielded less conclusive results, but may also be beneficial in preventing or delaying Alzheimer's and dementia symptoms.

Always talk to your doctor about possible medication interactions.

4: Mental stimulation

Those who continue learning new things throughout life and challenging their brains are less likely to develop Alzheimer's disease and dementia. In essence, you need to "use it or lose it."

In the groundbreaking NIH ACTIVE study, older adults who received as few as 10 sessions of mental training not only improved their cognitive functioning in daily activities in the months after the training, but continued to show long-lasting improvements 10 years later.

Activities involving multiple tasks or requiring communication, interaction, and organization offer the greatest protection. Set aside time each day to stimulate your brain:

Learn something new. Study a foreign language, practice a musical instrument, read the newspaper or a good book, or take up a new hobby. The greater the novelty and challenge, the greater the benefit.

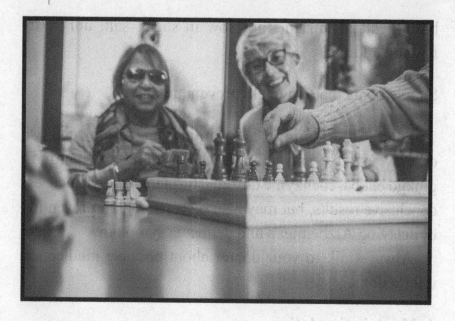

Practice memorization. Start with something short, progressing to something a little more involved, such as the 50 U.S. state capitals. Create rhymes and patterns to strengthen your memory connections.

Enjoy strategy games, puzzles, and riddles. Brain teasers and strategy games provide a great mental workout and build your capacity to form and retain cognitive associations. Do a crossword puzzle, play board games, cards, or word and number games such as Scrabble or Sudoku.

Practice the 5 Ws. Observe and report like a crime detective. Keep a "Who, What, Where, When, and Why" list of your daily experiences. Capturing visual details keeps your neurons firing.

Follow the road less traveled. Take a new route, eat with your non-dominant hand, and rearrange your computer file system. Vary your habits regularly to create new brain pathways.

5: Quality sleep

It's common for people with Alzheimer's disease to suffer from insomnia and other sleep problems. But new research suggests that disrupted sleep isn't just a symptom of Alzheimer's, but a possible risk factor.

An increasing number of studies have linked poor sleep to higher levels of beta-amyloid, a sticky brain-clogging protein that in turn further interferes with sleep—especially with the deep sleep necessary for memory formation. Other studies emphasize the importance of uninterrupted sleep for flushing out brain toxins.

If nightly sleep deprivation is slowing your thinking and affecting your mood, you may be at greater risk of developing symptoms of Alzheimer's disease. The vast majority of adults need at least 8 hours of sleep per night.

Sleep tips

Get screened for sleep apnea. If you've received complaints about your snoring, you may want to get tested for sleep apnea, a potentially dangerous condition where breathing is disrupted during sleep. Treatment can make a huge difference in both your health and sleep quality.

Establish a regular sleep schedule. Going to bed and getting up at the same time reinforces your natural circadian rhythms. Your brain's clock responds to regularity.

Be smart about napping. While taking a nap can be a great way to recharge, especially for older adults, it can make insomnia worse. If insomnia is a problem for you, consider eliminating napping. If you must nap, do it in the early afternoon, and limit it to thirty minutes.

Set the mood. Reserve your bed for sleep and sex, and ban television and computers from the bedroom (both are stimulating and may lead to difficulties falling asleep).

Create a relaxing bedtime ritual. Take a hot bath, do some light stretches, write in your journal, or dim the lights. As it becomes habit, your nightly ritual will send a powerful signal to your brain that it's time for deep restorative sleep.

Quiet your inner chatter. When stress, anxiety, or negative internal dialogues keep you awake, get out of bed. Try reading or relaxing in another room for twenty minutes, then hop back in.

6: Stress management

Chronic or persistent stress can take a heavy toll on the brain, leading to shrinkage in a key memory area, hampering nerve cell growth, and increasing the risk of Alzheimer's disease and dementia. Yet simple stress management tools can minimize its harmful effects.

Get your stress levels in check with these proven techniques

Breathe. Quiet your stress response with deep, abdominal breathing. Restorative breathing is powerful, simple, and free.

Schedule daily relaxation activities. Keeping stress under control requires regular effort. Make relaxation a priority, whether it's a walk in the park, playtime with your dog, yoga, or a soothing bath.

Nourish inner peace. Regular meditation, prayer, reflection, and religious practice may immunize you against the damaging effects of stress.

Make fun a priority. All work and no play is not good for your stress levels or your brain. Make time for leisure activities that bring you joy, whether it be stargazing, playing the piano, or working on your bike.

Keep your sense of humor. This includes the ability to laugh at yourself. The act of laughing helps your body fight stress.

Other tips to reduce the risk of Alzheimer's

Just as what's good for the body is also good for the brain, so too is the converse: what's bad for the body is bad for the brain.

Stop smoking. Smoking is one of the most preventable risk factors for Alzheimer's disease. One study found that smokers over the age of 65 have a nearly 80% higher risk of Alzheimer's than those who have never smoked. When you stop smoking, the brain benefits from improved circulation almost immediately.

Control blood pressure and cholesterol levels. Both high blood pressure and high total cholesterol are associated with an increased risk of Alzheimer's disease and vascular dementia. Improving those numbers are good for your brain as well as your heart.

Watch your weight. Extra pounds are a risk factor for Alzheimer's disease and other types of dementia. A major study found that people who were overweight in midlife were twice as likely to develop Alzheimer's down the line, and those who were obese had three times the risk. Losing weight can go a long way to protecting your brain.

Drink only in moderation. While there appear to be brain benefits in consuming red wine in moderation, heavy alcohol consumption can dramatically raise the risk of Alzheimer's and accelerate brain aging.

CHAPTER EIGHT

Treatment of Alzheimer's Disease

THE TREATMENT OF Alzheimer's disease can be placed under medication based and non-medication based categories.

A. Treatment With Drugs

FDA has classified two groups of pharmaceuticals for the treatment of this disease and these are cholinesterase inhibitors and partial glutamate antagonists.

But none of the drugs can perfectly slowdown the rate of progression of Alzheimer's disease. In patients suffering from this disorder, the process of formation of the brain neurotransmitter, especially the acetylcholine stops and research, has indicated that this chemical plays a crucial role in memory formation.

The cholinesterase inhibitors (ChEIs) participate in blocking the breakdown of this neurotransmitter and therefore, help in memory formation.

FDA has approved four cholinesterase inhibitors, namely donepezil hydrochloride, rivastigmine, galantamine and tacrine for the treatment of Alzheimer's disease but only the first three are used by the medical experts as the fourth one is risky and causes severe side effects.

Studies have clearly indicated that these drugs slow down the rate of disease progression only for about 6-12 months and then the disease starts advancing again.

FDA has approved the use of rivastigmine and galantamine for the treatment of mild and moderate symptoms of Alzheimer's disease but donepezil can be used for the treatment of mild, moderate and severe symptoms.

The exact reason why these two drugs are not used against the severe symptoms of the disease is not clear. The major side effects of ChEIs are associated with the gastrointestinal system and they include nausea, cramping, diarrhea and vomiting.

These symptoms can be controlled by changing the timing of medication as well as the intake of a small amount of food and about 75-90% of the patients have the potential of tolerating the therapeutic doses of cholinesterase inhibitors. Glutamate is the chief excitatory neurotransmitter of the brain.

One hypothesis suggests that excessive secretion of glutamate is harmful for the brain as it damages nerve cells.

Memantine is a drug that slows down the rate of activation of nerve cells by glutamate and therefore, reduces the progression of this disorder.

This drug can be used for treating both mild and severe disease. The patient recovers faster if a dose of cholinesterase inhibitors and memantine are given together.

Non-medication based treatments include orientation of the patient towards social activities like singing, dancing, walking etc. Cognitive rehabilitation may be helpful in this regard. The chief psychiatric symptoms associated with Alzheimer's disease are irritation, depression, hallucinations, anxiety and sleep disorders.

Although standard psychiatric drugs are used for the treatment of these symptoms, none of the drugs have been approved by the FDA. These symptoms become more intense as the disease advances so that treatment with medication becomes necessary. Agitation becomes more severe in the later stages of the disease.

Agitation is controlled by a number of agents for example, beta-blockers, anxiolytics, antipsychotics and mood stabilizing anticonvulsants. Newer antipsychotic drugs have taken the place of the older drugs and are giving fruitful results, for example, risperidone, clozapine and olanzapine.

Depression is another very common symptom of Alzheimer's disease and the patients can be treated with antidepressants, namely sertraline and citalopram. Anxiety in this disorder can be treated with benzodiazepines, for example, diazepam.

Non-benzodiazepines anxiolytics like buspirone are generally preferred for the treatment. Insomnia is another symptom that can crop up in patients of Alzheimer's disease at any part of their life.

Trazodone is a promising drug used for overcoming this symptom. A number of clinical research trials have been carried out by increasing or decreasing the amount of Aß1-42 but no successful result has been achieved.

Caring for the caregiver is an essential aspect while dealing with an Alzheimer's disease patient. Caregiving is a distressing experience and proper education of the caregiver is essential. The 3Rs, namely repeat, reassure and redirect can help a caregiver in reducing the troublesome behavior as well as limiting the use of medication in the patients.

The short-term training programs can help a caregiver to increase his or her confidence while dealing with the patients. Alzheimer's disease is a curse and it makes the condition of a person worse and death is the ultimate fate in later stages. Love, care and support can, however, help the patient to enjoy life.

Latest Drugs For Treating Alzheimer's Disease

Since Alzheimer's disease is commonly a slow process, the disease affects people differently and therefore individuals respond to different treatments uniquely.

Currently, there is no drug or treatment program that stops the progression of Alzheimer's disease. However, for individuals who are in the mild and middle stages of the disease, certain drugs have proven successful.

The latest drugs for treating Alzheimer's disease are:

Aricept (donepezil) *taking Now*

Given orally, this medication is a reversible inhibitor of the enzyme acetylcholinesterase. It is used to treat symptoms in people with mild to moderate Alzheimer's disease. Our brains normally produce acetylcholine, a chemical thought to be important for learning and memory. People with Alzheimer's disease have lower brain levels of acetylcholine.

Aricept acts by decreasing the activity of acetylcholinesterase, an enzyme whose function is to break down acetylcholine. It is believed that by reducing the breakdown of acetylcholine, it will lead to an increase in the level of acetylcholine in the brain.

Cognex (tacrine)

Given orally, this is another medication that inhibits the enzyme acetylcholinesterase. Tacrine will not cure Alzheimer's disease, and it will not stop the disease from getting worse. However, tacrine can improve thinking ability in some patients with Alzheimer's disease.

Exelon (rivastigmine)

Another cholinesterase inhibitor given orally. This medication is used to treat loss of memory and thinking ability associated with Alzheimer's disease.

Razadyne (galantamine)

This medication was formerly known as Reminyl. It was changed to razadyne on July 1st, 2005. Razadyne is a competitive acetylcholinesterase inhibitor. It has been shown to treat some of the symptoms of Alzheimer's disease successfully.

Namenda (memantine)

Approved by the FDA in October, 2003, this medication is given orally, and works different from the acetylcholinesterase inhibitors. Glutamate is the main excitatory neurotransmitter in the brain. It it thought that too much glutamate in the brain can cause cellular damage. Namenda works by blocking the effects of glutamate.

Antioxidants

Clinical trials have shown that vitamin E slows the progression of Alzheimer's disease by about seven months. Current clinical trials are underway to determine whether vitamin E will slow the progression of Alzheimer's disease.

Other clinical trials are underway to determine whether vitamin E and selenium supplements can help slow or prevent symptoms of Alzheimer's disease.

Ginkgo Biloba

The latest studies using Ginkgo Biloba extract from leaves has shown this chemical to be of some help with treating Alzheimer's disease symptoms. However, there is no evidence that Ginkgo Biloba will cure or prevent Alzheimer's disease. Currently, there is some clinical evidence showing that Ginkgo Biloba can delay cognitive deficits or prevent dementia to a certain extent in older people.

Estrogen

Clinical trials have been conducted showing that estrogen therapy can protect the brain against damages caused by Alzheimer's disease. These studies were originally conducted using estrogen on women for hormone replacement therapy. A positive response regarding Alzheimer's disease prevention was noted as a side effect.

Current evidence has shown that while estrogen therapy can help prevent the severity or symptoms of Alzheimer's disease, it will not slow the progression of Alzheimer's disease once it has already been diagnosed.

B. Treatment With Food

1. Curry

Curry is the Indian favor which is eaten daily and contains curcumin that helps to trigger the production of enzymes protecting against any oxidative disease. It also is filled with phenols, the natural inflammation fighter.

2. Garlic

Garlic is one of nature's superfoods that contains allicin that helps to strengthen the immune system fighting against any harmful toxins and micro-organism naturally. It also contains iron that helps in producing red blood cells and improving circulation of the blood to brain cells.

3. Dark green leaf juice

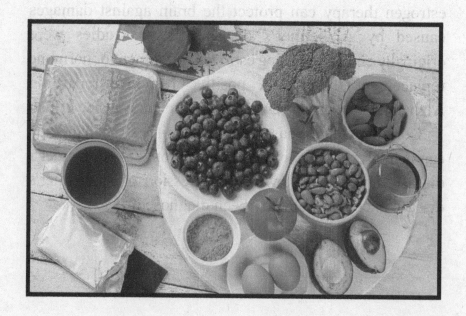

Dark green leaf juice contains hundreds of phytochemicals that help to detoxify our body from free radical build-up, removing heavy metals from our brain and have an anti-virus, anti-bacteria, immune boosting resulting in anti-inflammation. It also helps to strengthen the liver, the vital organ for our body's detoxification. Dark green leaf juice is best for detoxification against any plague and tangle in our body.

4. Cold water fish

Cold water fish contains high amounts of fatty acids Omega 3 and 6 that help to lower the levels of bad cholesterol and triglyceride resulting in a healthy heart and improved blood circulation.

5. Cinnamon powder

One the most powerful natural superfoods. Contains essential oils that help to strengthen the immune system caused by virus and bacteria and infection caused by wound. Studies show that cinnamon also will help to regulate levels of glucose in the bloodstream which aids blood circulation.

6. Tomato

Tomato contains high amounts of beta carotene, the powerful antioxidant that helps to remove toxins from our body and fight against free radicals building up in our brain. Beta carotene in tomato is tough to digest. Be sure to take it with vitamin C to increase the absorption.

7. Grape juice

Grape juice contains high amounts of iron that helps the production of red blood cells resulting in increased oxygen levels in the blood stream for brain cells.

8. Broccoli

Broccoli contains high amounts of vitamin C and fiber that helps to strengthen the immune system and reduce cholesterol building up in the arteries, increasing the blood circulation to brain vessels.

In fact, any foods that contain high amounts of antioxidants resulting in winning the battle of free radical build up in our body, including our brain, will help to prevent and treat Alzheimer's disease.

C. Treatment With vitamins and Minerals

1. Vitamin complex

Vitamin complex is supportive for people with Alzheimer's disease, a disorder that is also associated with low levels of pyridoxine and cobalamin. Vitamins B5, B6, B12 are vital for strengthening the immune system fighting against free radicals building up in certain brain areas.

2. Iron

The right amount of iron will help the production of red blood cells and improve circulation of blood as well as oxygen levels in the blood stream, which is vital for brain cells that need better function.

3. Vitamin C

Vitamin C is an antioxidant vitamin. It helps to strengthen our immune system in fighting off the early formation of free radicals and DNA mutation. Our body cannot produce vitamin C. Fruits and vegetables contain high quantities of vitamin C such as kiwi, broccoli, lemon, and apple.

4. Vitamin E

Vitamin E helps to strengthen the immune system and restore the balance of hormones.

5. Zinc

Zinc not only helps prostate gland increase production of fluid and semen, but also helps to promote the production of testosterone by stopping the production of procalin and reduce the binding of the sex hormone binding globulin. Increasing the testosterone levels in men will help to prevent and treat Alzheimer's disease.

6. Magnesium

Magnesium and potassium helps to strengthen and prevent calcium forming the arterial wall. The right amounts of magnesium, potassium and calcium not only help in increasing blood circulation but will also lower high blood pressure. Calcium deficiency may cause the loss of memory and senility.

D. Treatment With Herbs

1. Ginko biloba

Ginko biloba enhances the circulation to the central nervous system and has a tendency to stabilize abnormal nerve communication in the brain. It also is a powerful antioxidant that helps to protect the brain cells from free radical damage.

2. Korean ginseng

Korean ginseng contains ginsenosides which is an anti-stress remedy. It also helps to increase protein synthesis and improves the performance of neurotransmitters in the brain, resulting in curbing the onset of psychological deterioration and aiding mental condition.

3. Huperzine A

Huperzia, as it is now called, contains a wide variety of alkaloids, including lycodoline, lycoclavine, and serratinine that help to increase the acetylcholine activity in the brain resulting in improved memory and behavior problems.

4. Kut

The mixture of herbal formula in Japan also helps in increasing the activity of acetycholine in the cortex and hippocampus section of the brain and stimulating the growth of nerve cells.

5. Garlic Extract

Garlic extract helps to improve the immune system and blood circulation in our body as well as preventing the formation of free radicals.

6. Pumpkin seed

Pumpkin seeds contains high amounts of zinc and iron. Zinc is a vital mineral for a healthy prostate gland which helps to trigger the production of free testosterone. Iron helps the reproduction of red blood cells and increases the oxygen levels in the blood stream that is essential for brain cells.

7. Chlorella

Chlorella contains the antioxidant, chlorophyll, that helps to protect against the formation of free radicals and improves the circulation of blood in our body. Studies show that chlorella also helps to protect brain cells caused by high levels of stress hormones. The nucleic acid in chlorella also helps to improve memory.

E. With conventional approach

1. Inflammation

Strengthening the immune system will help to fight off foreign substances, molecules as well as the formation of free radicals that help to decrease or prevent any degree of inflammation in joints, skin, and the brain resulting in skin wrinkle, arthritis and memory problems. Cinnamon powder contain high amounts of antioxidant beta carotene that can help to strengthen your immune system and fight against any inflammation.

2. Mini-Stroke

Mini stroke may not have any impact in brain cells but hundreds or thousands of mini strokes may cause the blockage of brain vessels resulting in the accumulation of plagues and tangles.

Therefore, taking life style changes to protect overall health may help to prevent or delay any other memory loss and symptoms of Alzheimer's disease. Garlic contains high amounts of iron that help to reproduce blood cells as well improve oxygen levels resulting in better circulation of blood to brain cells.

3. Control high blood pressure

High blood pressure causes the heart to work harder to provide oxygen to brain cells resulting in plague building up in the arterial wall and hardening of arteries. Chlorella contains chlorophyll that helps not only to remove plague from the arterial wall, but also heavy metals that have accumulated in our brain.

4. Control levels of cholesterol

Cholesterol causes the clogging of brain vessels. Fish contains high amounts of fatty acid Omega 3 and 6 help to inhibit blood clotting that causes a serious blockage in the vessels of the brain.

5. Eating more vegetable and fruits

Vegetable and fruits contain antioxidant vitamins and other photochemicals that can help to protect brain cells from damage from free radicals and stop the progression of brain cells dying off due to Alzheimer's disease. Others such as reducing the intake of alcohol, stopping smoking, getting regular exercise and staying mentally active also help as well.

F. Treatment With supplements

1. Melatonin

As we age, the production of melatonin in the pineal gland diminishes. The intake of a melatonin supplement may exert a powerful antioxidant activity that easily helps to prevent the formation of cell radicals in our body including the brain.

2. Carnosine

Carnosine helps to block the formation of glycosylation, caused by sugar aldehydes reacting with the amino acid on the protein molecule. It also helps to remove toxic chemicals such as copper and zinc from the brain.

3. DHEA

DHEA is a hormone produced by the adrenal gland that helps to regulate the balance of our body's hormones. A deficiency of DHEA causes hormone imbalance in men as well as women. Studies show that an intake of DHEA is necessary for aging men for improving mental ability and alleviating stress.

4. Coenezyme Q 10

Coenezyme Q 10 helps to increase the circulation and oxygen levels of the blood stream as we know that lack of oxygen in the blood can exacerbate cognitive deterioration.

5. Lecithin

Choline and inositol in the lecithin helps to increase production of acetylcholine in our body, thereby helping the communication and signal-transmission between brain cells. An increase in lecithin will prompt brain cells to produce more acetylcholine, thus improving memory.

6. Taurine

Besides helping to protect the formation of free radicals in brain cells and enhance nervous cell function, taurine is essential in protecting the supply of magnesium and calcium in the brain.

CHAPTER NINE

Powerful Natural Remedies for
Dementia and Alzheimer's

DEMENTIA AND ALZHEIMER'S are truly horrible and cruel diseases. But new research is showing that you cannot only 100% prevent them from occurring, but you can actually reverse their effects.

Here's 10 of the best natural remedies and treatments for dementia and Alzheimer's according to the experts.

Dementia is such a shocking disease. Because the mental and behavioural changes happen so gradually in a sufferer, you're left to watch your loved one slowly deteriorate before your eyes and you grieve every time they take a turn for the worst.

Can Natural Remedies Help to Treat and Even Reverse Dementia?

The answer to this question is a definite yes. You just need to start treating the affected person as soon as possible (the earlier the better). But even if they are in the latter stages of the disease, you can still help them tremendously by using natural therapies.

In fact, you won't believe the astounding changes that will happen, even within a few short weeks. And the best part about using natural remedies for treating dementia over pharmaceutical medications is that there are no harmful side effects.

All of these natural and home remedies are safe. You have nothing to lose by trying them, so let's get started with our top 10 recommendations in order of importance...

Natural Remedies for Dementia and Alzheimer's Treatment Option #1: Coconut Oil...

Coconut oil works so incredibly well for dementia patients that it almost seems like a "magic bullet" cure. Coconut oil contains substances called ketones, which are a powerful brain food (one of the best actually). The healthy fats contained in coconut oil also help to rebuild the lining of the nerves so brain communication is increased and healthy nerve function is enhanced.

Virtually all dementia suffers (especially Alzheimer's and Parkinson's patients) who try it receive overwhelmingly positive benefits. I had the privilege of interviewing world-renowned coconut oil expert and author, Dr Bruce Fife, not so long ago and he spoke extensively about the power of coconut oil for preventing and reversing Alzheimer's disease (and backed it up with some very reputable studies).

Here's a snippet of what Dr Fife had to say in that interview…

Coconut ketone therapy has the potential to stop the progression of Alzheimer's, reverse it, and in some cases, completely eliminate the disease.

The medical research on coconut oil derived ketone therapy is remarkable. In one study, for example, Alzheimer's patients were split into two groups. Each group was given a beverage to drink. The beverage given to one group contained MCFAs from coconut oil, the other beverage contained the types of fatty acids ordinarily found in the diet.

Ninety minutes later, the investigators had the patients take cognitive and memory tests. The results showed that those patients that consumed the beverage with MCFAs scored significantly higher on the tests.

This study was remarkable for three primary reasons. First, it demonstrated that MCFAs do have a positive effect on Alzheimer's patients. This is incredible because no drug currently in use has shown a positive effect like this.

The very best that Alzheimer's drugs can do is to slightly slow down the progression of the disease. None have ever been able to stop it or even produce any improvement. MCFAs showed actual improvement.

Second, the results of the MCFAs were seen almost immediately: just ninety minutes after taking the drink, the patients showed measurable improvement on test scores.

Third, the improvement was seen after only one dose of MCFAs. The patients didn't need to take hundreds of doses of a drug for months at a time to see any benefit, the benefit was measureable after a single dose. There is no drug on the market that can come close to matching the effects that Alzheimer's patients can get from coconut oil.

How Much Coconut Oil Do You Need to Take?

Firstly, understand that you cannot overdose on coconut oil… ever. However, too much in the beginning can cause mild diarrhea in some people so it's best to start off slowly and gradually build up. Two tablespoons taken three times daily in divided doses (with food) is best to begin with.

After a few weeks, you can then increase to four tablespoons consumed three times per day. Just make sure the coconut oil you buy is 100% organic, virgin coconut oil. Processed coconut oil contains trans fatty acids and should never be eaten.

In addition to taking coconut oil every day, it's also a good idea to make up some coconut milk and use this instead of drinking cow's milk. Processed dairy is exceptionally bad for dementia suffers (and should be avoided completely), but coconut milk is exceptionally good. You can find out how to easily make your own coconut milk here… wellnessmama.com

1: Cinnamon Extract

Researchers have now been able to confirm that dementia diseases such as Alzheimer's are actually a form of diabetes. In fact, Alzheimer's is now being labelled as type III diabetes. What this means is that the brain has basically become "insulin resistant".

But what's really exciting is that cinnamon extract, which works extremely well for type I and type II diabetes, also works very well for dementia – especially Alzheimer's disease...

In a study published in the Journal of Alzheimer's Disease, researchers found two compounds in cinnamon extract that help to stop the disintegration and dysfunction of the tau protein.

By keeping this protein strong, scientists believe neurofibrillary tangles (these "tangles" are thought to be a prime suspect and cause in brain disorders such as Alzheimer's disease) can be prevented and even reversed.

Insulin and insulin receptors located in the brain are also essential for memory and cognitive functions, and these have been found to be significantly lower in Alzheimer's patients. But cinnamon regulates brain insulin activity, which in turn, helps to restore normal brain functioning.

2: The Right Type of Cinnamon...

Make sure you only ever use cinnamon extract or cinnamon bark extract (capsules or powder) that come from Ceylon (Sri Lanka). Do not buy cheap cinnamon such as cassia or any products that contain this type of cinnamon. It won't work anywhere near as well.

Take a heaped teaspoon of cinnamon powder three times daily with or without meals and use it in your cooking as much as possible. You can also make up a delicious cinnamon and ginger tea for an extra supply if you wish (ginger is also very good for dementia). With the capsules, a total of 3 grams daily (or more) will be required for best results.

3: B Group Vitamins, Vitamin D and Vitamin E

A study published in Proceedings of the National Academy of Sciences revealed the B group vitamins, in particular, vitamin B6, B12 and folic acid, can help slow the progression of Alzheimer's disease. What was stated in the article is quite exciting for dementia sufferers as well as those wanting to prevent the disease.

"The fact that B-family vitamins may play a significant role in dementia, or more specifically in warding it off, has been consistently illustrated.

What is news from the current study, however, is that high-dose B-vitamin treatment in people at risk for the disease 'slowed shrinkage of whole brain volume,' and especially reduced shrinkage in areas known to be affected in Alzheimer's disease."

Vitamin B3 (niacin) and vitamin B6 are needed by the body to form neurotransmitters, making them crucial for the health and correct functioning of the nervous system and brain. B12 is essential for the production of a substance known as myelin, the white sheath that surrounds nerve fibers.

The B group vitamins, especially folic acid, also help to reduce homocysteine levels in the body, another major precursor of dementia and dementia related diseases.

A vitamin D deficiency has been repeatedly linked to brain problems such as poor memory and recall attainability. Researchers believe that vitamin D protects brain cells and may even be able to help damaged neurons regenerate.

Vitamin D is also a strong anti-inflammatory and immune boosting nutrient. Because inflammation and low immunity are such powerful factors in the onset and development of dementia diseases, vitamin D could quite possibly be the most important and crucial nutrient for all dementia sufferers.

Vitamin E, on the other hand, has also been found to prevent and even treat dementia diseases such as Alzheimer's. In fact, 60 years ago in the animal industry, farmers were actually able to prevent and cure Alzheimer's disease in animals by feeding them high doses of vitamin E.

Then, after human studies on vitamin E and Alzheimer's disease some 30 years later (we're obviously a little slower to catch up), the University of California and the Salk Institute came out and said... "Vitamin E can ease memory loss in Alzheimer's patients."

Best Sources of B Group Vitamins, Vitamin D and Vitamin E

For vitamin B12, a sublingual spray containing methylcobalamin is the absolute best and most absorbable way to get your daily dose (a few sprays under the tongue and you're done). Here's what one looks like... B12 Sublingual

Spray. For the other B group vitamins (and an extra dose of B12), a good quality B complex supplement will suffice.

There are two ways to get your vitamin D,. Firstly, get out in the sun. 20-40 minutes of regular sun exposure a day (depending on the temperature), is still the best way to receive the vitamin D your body needs.

The most important areas of exposure are the face and back of the hands. In addition to this, and especially if you live in cold climates, supplementation with vitamin D3 (the same as what the sun makes), is crucial.

The best sources are vitamin D3 supplements and cod liver oil. Just remember too, our bodies need lots of vitamin D so don't be afraid of overdosing on this vital nutrient (vitamin D expert, Dr Cedric Garland, recommends a minimum of 5000 IU's of vitamin D per day so I suggest you follow his guidelines and not the RDA).

For vitamin E, the best source is without a doubt unprocessed red palm oil. The benefit of red palm oil is not only is it incredibly high in the eight different forms of molecules categorized as vitamin E (including the "king of kings" alpha-tocopherol), it's also high in the healthy ketone fats all dementia sufferers need.

And in addition, red palm oil helps with blood circulation, along with providing powerful neuroprotection just for good measure.

Even Dr Oz says red palm oil is a miracle oil for longevity so start getting some into you or your loved one as soon as you can.

4: Minerals

Minerals are commonly referred to as "the sparks of life". They are what keep our body battery going and keep it charged. Minerals are also needed by the brain's "electrical circuit" to function properly. You may not know this but your brain is one incredible and very intricate circuit board.

Every time you think a thought (or every time your brain is at work is probably a better description), little "sparks" and electrical currents are busy racing and crisscrossing each other in a dazzling and spectacular light show. In fact, while your brain's at work it's actually producing enough electricity to power a light bulb.

So, how it basically works is when you think a thought, that particular thought is then transferred or relayed to the area of the brain that needs it by "sparks" or electricity. And minerals are one of the crucial components that make this all happen and make the process run smoothly.

But when your brain lacks the minerals it needs for this process to work correctly, these sparks begin to "jump" in the wrong places. Or even worse, they don't jump at all. This is the beginnings and eventual progression of diseases such as Alzheimer's.

How to Continuously Replenish the Brain (And Body) With These Essential Nutrients...

Our bodies need over 60 essential minerals and trace elements every day to function correctly and at its peak.

Exactly how many minerals our brain needs to function properly, no one really knows. But it's lots.

Magnesium is one of the most important minerals for the brain and for healthy nerve function (this is also one mineral that's severely lacking from our modern day diets). Studies have shown that dementia sufferers can improve, some quite dramatically in fact, from correct mineral supplementation.

Liquid colloidal minerals are the best and most absorbable way to get the required 60+ minerals your body and brain needs every day (they're the only way really).

For magnesium, a transdermal magnesium spray is the best way to go. Magnesium is tough for the body to absorb but with a transdermal magnesium spray, it's penetrated directly into the blood stream via the skin.

If this is not practical or you don't like the idea of spraying an oil on your skin every day, there is a terrific magnesium supplement available called Natural Calm, which is actually one of the very few oral magnesium supplements on the market that's highly absorbable (and doesn't taste awful). You can check it out here if you're interested... Natural Calm.

5: Omega-3s

Omega-3 fatty acids are yet another fat that are incredibly healthy for the brain and nervous system. They contain the EPA and DHA essential fatty acids, which help to prevent brain cell damage and keep the nervous system in peak working order.

And they don't just help to slow down the progression of dementia diseases such as Alzheimer's and Parkinson's either, they also help to lower ones risk of developing the disease in the first place.

The best sources of omega-3s are fish oil, cod liver oil and krill oil. Krill oil is probably the pick of the bunch because it contains a substance called Astaxanthin, which is a potent "brain food" and has been shown in studies to help prevent neurodegeneration of the brain.

6: Build-Up the Immune System

This is probably one of the most overlooked remedies and treatments for dementia. Stamford University have discovered that boosting the body's immune system can help with Alzheimer's disease. Here's what was stated in an article published in the UK's, The Telegraph...

"Alzheimer's could be prevented and even cured by boosting the brain's own immune response, new research suggests. Researchers at Stanford University discovered that nerve cells die because cells (known as microglial cells), which are supposed to clear the brain of bacteria, viruses and dangerous deposits, stop working".

This makes perfect sense, since bacteria, viruses and "dangerous deposits" such as mercury and aluminium have now been vindicated as prime suspects in the onset and development of diseases such as Alzheimer's.

In fact, researchers from Umea University found that the herpes simplex virus increases the risk of Alzheimer's disease. They said... "Our results clearly show that there is a link between infections of herpes simplex virus and the risk of developing Alzheimer's disease".

So, building up the body's immune system and keeping these microglial cells healthy and in tip top condition is absolutely vital for the prevention and reversal of dementia, particularly in regards to Alzheimer's disease.

7: Chlorella and Borax...

It's no secret (at least in the natural health circles) that an accumulation of heavy metals in the brain, particularly mercury, aluminium, lead and fluoride, are one of the major causes of dementia. These heavy metals trigger what's commonly known as "brain drain."

Heavy metal toxicity also wreaks havoc on the body's nervous system, which is why diseases such as Parkinson's, Huntington's and motor neuron disease have been linked to heavy metal accumulation.

So, the flushing out (chelation) of these heavy metals from the nervous system and brain is definitely a top priority for the prevention and treatment of dementia.

And the two best ways to accomplish this is through the supplementation of a stunning superfood called chlorella and Borax powder (yes, I know it's classed as an ant killer but stay with me on this one).

Chlorella is a powerful detoxifier, probably the most powerful yet discovered in fact. It has a unique ability to pull heavy metals out of the body but leave the good minerals (essential minerals) alone. Chlorella also removes other toxic poisons, chemicals and pesticides from the digestive tract so they don't enter the bloodstream and poison the body.

A Russian study found that chlorella, combined with cilantro (coriander), was able to remove all heavy metals from the body, including mercury, with no adverse side effects. These remarkable benefits make chlorella the #1 detox food available, followed closely by Borax.

Borax can also be used to remove heavy metals from the body, including the brain and nervous system. Walter Last, in his ground-breaking chapter on Borax as an arthritis cure, makes mention of using borax to remove heavy metals from the body, particularly fluoride (which is incredibly toxic to the brain), safely and effectively.

Borax (boron) is also very effective at balancing hormone levels in both men and women. According to famed author and medical doctor, Dr Mark Hyman, hormone imbalances are another major cause of dementia.

Now, in case you don't already know, Borax is actually used as a food preservative so don't be scared off by it.

8: Cholesterol

For years now, we've been told that cholesterol is bad for us and if we eat too much, we'll end up dropping dead of a heart attack. Well this information is totally false.

And thankfully, the truth on this one is finally coming out. So many articles (such as this one) are finally relaying the real facts, that eating cholesterol containing foods doesn't cause heart disease, and that cholesterol actually helps to prevent and treat dementia and Alzheimer's.

Think about this... your brain by weight is 75% pure cholesterol. And the insulating material that surrounds your brain is actually 100% pure cholesterol. Without enough cholesterol, this "insulation" begins to shrink, which also causes your brain to shrink.

Remember what I said about minerals and the brain's electrical circuit board? You can ask any qualified electrician about this... if you don't insulate electrical wires or currents then the electricity is basically free to "jump" wherever it pleases (this is why electrical wires are always wrapped in rubber or plastic; it gives insulation). Well, your brain is exactly the same.

Without enough insulation (cholesterol), your brain's electrical currents (sparks) aren't going to hit their mark, so to speak. The result? Neurological problems and diseases such as Alzheimer's. This is another reason why cholesterol lowering drugs are so dangerous and are actually one of the causes of Alzheimer's disease.

So be sure you or your loved one get enough cholesterol every day by taking some cod liver oil and eating at least two eggs each day, along with eating plenty of cold water fish, shellfish, natural butter, red meat (including the fat) and chicken with the skin on.

9: Foods to Avoid Foods to Eat

Certain foods definitely help with the prevention and treatment of dementia, while other foods are guaranteed to make this condition much worse.

The foods and liquids you should be eating and drinking more of are the staples. These include...

Filtered water – Helps to flush toxins from the body and hydrate the cells (including brain cells).

Green tea or Matcha tea – Both contain powerful antioxidants known as catechins which remove harmful toxins and chemicals from the body. A component in these teas has also been shown to decrease brain beta-amyloid plaque formation.

Turmeric, Ginger, Cinnamon, Black pepper, Chilli's (Cayenne pepper), Rosemary, Coriander and Garlic – All of these herbs and spices are potent anti-viral, anti-inflammatory and immune boosting foods (everything dementia sufferers need).

Reishi and Cordyceps mushrooms – Both are immune boosting and contain strong neuro-protective properties.

Probiotics – Needed for healthy gut function, which in turn produces healthy brain function and healthy immunity. You can learn how to make your own fermented foods such as kefir, sauerkraut, kombucha and yoghurt here... Cultures for Health.

Whole foods – Eating plenty of organic mixed berries, green leafy vegetables, liver (if you can stomach it), nuts and seeds such as chia and flaxseeds is vital. When it comes to buying these, fresh is definitely best.

For the foods you should be avoiding or not eating at all, here's the top ones...

Margarine – This is a man-made death food that's guaranteed to fry your brain and make brain disorders such as dementia much worse. Don't touch it with a ten foot pole.

Refined (processed) sugars – Makes your blood sticky and restricts circulation to areas of the brain. Another man-altered death food.

Gluten – Has been repeatedly linked to brain disorders and learning disabilities so all gluten containing foods are best avoided.

Trans fats – Margarine, all baked goods, fast food and vegetable oils, (especially the ones that you find sitting on the shelf in supermarkets in clear bottles), are full of brain damaging trans fats and free radicals. These must all be completely avoided if you want to prevent or reverse dementia.

Processed dairy – Pasteurized milk, cheese, cream and yoghurts are toxic gunk that stick to the lining of the gut and prevent the absorption of nutrients. Unless you have access to unpasteurized dairy products, use alternatives such as coconut milk or almond milk.

10: Stay Active (Physically and Mentally)

Remaining mentally and physically active has been well proven to not only delay the onset of dementia, but also help to improve the symptoms and even reverse the disease.

When it comes to using your brain, the old saying, "You Snooze You Lose" is definitely true. If you don't keep your body active it will eventually become stiff and seize up on you, and your brain is no different.

So you must keep it active and working. There's a direct correlation between mental stimulation, such as learning something new or doing puzzles, and a decreased risk of dementia and Alzheimer's.

Researchers believe mental challenges help to build up the brain, and by doing this, make it less prone to developing the lesions that can cause Alzheimer's disease. What's more, mental stimulation also helps to delay brain deterioration in people who already have the disease, and in many cases, can even reverse it.

Staying physically active is also crucial for delaying and improving the onset and development of dementia and has been well documented. Regular moderate exercise, such as walking, swimming, cycling, tai-chi or yoga, have all been associated with better retention of cognitive skills. However, the best form of exercise for dementia is weight training.

So, there you have our top 10 natural remedies for successfully treating and reversing dementia and Alzheimer's disease. But don't forget (no pun intended), that these remedies and recommendations are also exactly what you need to be taking and following to prevent dementia from ever affecting you. (Prevention is always best). And like we said earlier, you have nothing to lose by trying these treatments.

We recommend you start with Number 1 and then work your way down the list, using and utilizing as many of the remedies as you or your loved one can.

Expect to see some big results within 3-6 months. It will, however, take at least 12 months for a full recovery (or as close to a full recovery as you are going to get), so you must be patient and consistent with the daily application of these recommendations.

CHAPTER TEN

Coping with the Signs and Symptoms

THERE'S NO DOUBT about it. If someone you love develops Alzheimer's disease, your lives will be changed forever.

It's truly devastating to watch someone you love as they begin to lose their memory, and as the disease progresses, it also becomes a lot more difficult to care for that person. Let's take a look at a few basic ways in which you can cope more effectively as your loved one develops Alzheimer's.

The first step is to always find out everything you can about Alzheimer's disease, so that you know what it is, and how it's likely to progress. The more you know, the better prepared you will be for all potential eventualities.

It also makes it easier to understand exactly what your loved one is going through, so that you can be more supportive. Knowledge helps you to cope. If there's a support group in your area, you might want to join it, because shared experiences make it easier to cope with the situation.

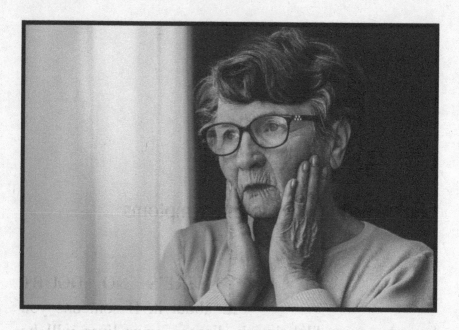

You may find that many of the other members can give you helpful advice and ideas about your situation, because they've already experienced similar things to what you're now going through. If you can't find a local group, try searching online, as there are support groups available on the Internet as well.

Many people with Alzheimer's fluctuate throughout the day. So try and establish a pattern of behavior - when is the condition most severe, and when is it least obvious? If you find there is a pattern, then you can plan your day to fit around that.

If you have a window of opportunity to get things done, then do them, so that you can concentrate on what you need to do, rather than worrying about your loved one.

You also need to start planning. Initially, it may be possible for you to care for your loved one at home, despite the Alzheimer's, but that may not always be the case. The reality is that Alzheimer's is degenerative, and over time, the condition will worsen. Medication may slow the progress of the disease, but it can't stop it.

Coping for someone with Alzheimer's is a huge emotional and financial burden, and it's important to make sure that you look after yourself as well.

The more prepared you are for the future, the easier it will be to deal with it when it arrives. Spend some time checking with your insurance agency, medicare and any other relevant organizations so that you're aware of what financial support you have available.

If you're finding it too hard to care for your loved one on your own, then look into the option of some form of adult daycare. It's important to research any facility you're considering as thoroughly as you can, so that you're comfortable that your loved one will be well cared for there while you take a break.

Unfortunately Alzheimer's is difficult to cope with, and the task can be draining emotionally, physically and financially. The important thing is that you're not alone; many thousands of families are struggling day to day with the same issues you're facing.

Find a way of balancing the needs of your loved one and your own needs, so that you don't wear yourself out in the process. Finally, make sure you spend some time remembering how much your loved one means to you, and never give up.

If you are providing care for someone with dementia, it is important to honor and recognize your own feelings of frustration and helplessness. However, when you feel frustrated, it is also important that you learn to express that feeling appropriately and ask for help when you need it. You must also take care of yourself and make time for yourself. Seek outside support to help you through the process.

Even if you are not the primary caregiver for someone with dementia, trying to communicate with them can still be a frustrating experience. Patients with dementia understand what you say in the context of their own world.

Trying to convince them that their world is incorrect or "not real" can make matters worse. Instead, it helps to remain calm and be sensitive to what they perceive to be reality.

You can prevent some forms of dementia, such as dementia due to a vitamin B-1 deficiency, by ensuring that you eat a nutritious, balanced diet.

You may also be able to prevent vascular dementia by taking good care of your heart with the help of your physician. And if you are diabetic, controlling your diabetes is critical. In many cases, though, there is no sure-fire way to prevent dementia.

A recent study at the Mayo clinic indicates that people who do not have psychiatric problems but who score very high on a personality test's pessimism scale have a

30 percent increased risk of developing dementia several decades later.

The same holds true for those people who score very high on the depression scale of personality test. For people who score high in both anxiety and pessimism, the risk of developing dementia later in life rises to 40 percent or more. So, developing a positive attitude and getting help if you suffer from depression may be helpful.

Doctors also recommend keeping your mind sharp by reading, writing stories, playing games, or starting a new hobby. Staying connected with friends and family also helps stimulate your memory and mental processes.

Living with a person with dementia

Helping someone going through this is something that all those close to them can be part of. It needn't be left only to the 'nearest and dearest' -good neighbours, colleagues and friends can all support and offer much needed friendship. Many families feel awkward and embarrassed because they have someone with dementia in the family.

They may feel cut off from other people and think that knowing about the dementia should be kept within the family circle. Ideally it is better that the person with dementia retains outside friendships and interests, helping them to keep a sense of their own identity and their place in their community.

Quite apart from the benefits to the individual of maintaining these contacts, carers need the breaks that seeing non-family members gives them. It's also vital that the person with dementia has short periods of time away from their family, which may be more possible early on in the dementia.

There will be times in the future when you may need to spend longer time together as care becomes more necessary. The relationship of the person with dementia to those who offer care will also change, especially if they are their spouse.

Their children will possibly become their carers, therefore reversing roles. The person with dementia may want to protect their family from their concerns, but also the children will begin to feel more protective towards their parent, as their capacity to manage daily life becomes less.

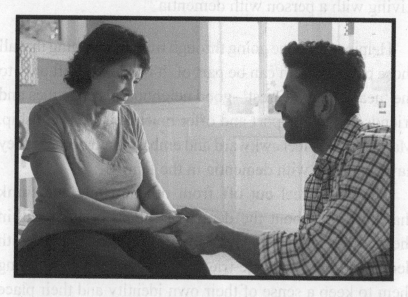

Above all, don't be tempted to think that all contacts must involve some kind of activity or purposeful task. Sometimes, the most vital moments can be when we simply sit and listen, or chat about shared experiences and enjoy each other's company, offering true friendship.

The key to being a good friend in these circumstances is to remain patient, flexible and attentive - not to mind the inevitable mood swings or difficulties that will arise.

Trying to keep things normal

Maintaining a sense of normality and familiarity is crucial, although easier said than done. They need to feel that life is going on the usual way as much as possible - that their company and their thoughts are as valued and respected as they ever were.

Above all, remember dementia affects a person's thinking, reasoning and memory, but that person's feelings remain intact. In the earlier stages, they may well want to talk about their fears and anxieties with both family and close friends.

Being willing to listen honestly is perhaps the greatest gift anyone can give to another in these circumstances and should not be under-valued. Listen to their plans for the future, it may not be comfortable but it is important that the person with dementia can feel as in control of their lives as possible.

Dementia can be a cruel and humiliating condition if not handled with care and understanding. Helping someone cope with it requires kindness and patience - qualities we all have to offer.

CHAPTER ELEVEN

Preventing and Slowing the Progression of Dementia

WALKING EVEN AS little as 1 1/2 hours per week at a pace of 21 to 30 minutes per mile is associated with improved cognitive function and decreased cognitive decline.

There is no known way to prevent dementia. However, there are actions that you can take to reduce your risk for dementia and, in some cases, slow the progression of the disease. These factors include:

- Exercise
- Diet
- Heart healthy behaviors
- Avoiding head injury

- Mental activities
- Socializing

Some factors may decrease the effect of the damage by developing more connections between the remaining brain cells, rather than preventing damage. With more connections between brain cells, function can be maintained longer despite damage to the brain.

Diet

A diet that includes a lot of fruit, vegetables, and whole grains may reduce the risk of developing dementia. These foods appear to protect brain neurons from chemicals, called free radicals, that damage cells. The protective chemicals in these foods are called antioxidants. Other foods that may protect against dementia include curcumin, the main ingredient in the spice tumeric, and omega-3 fatty acids, found in fish.

Exercise

Exercise leads to a healthier brain, just as it leads to better health for the rest of the body. Exercise and physical activity improve cognitive performance and reduce cognitive decline. The amount of exercise does not have to be extreme.

Research has found that moderate activity levels (for example, exercising just three times a week) decrease the risk of developing dementia. The effect is increased with a greater variety of activities and there appears to be a benefit, even if exercise is started late in life.

Keep Your Heart Healthy

The same factors that protect against heart disease help reduce some of the risk factors for dementia. These include, in addition to exercising and healthy eating, not smoking, maintaining a healthy weight, controlling blood pressure, relaxing and reducing stress.

Mental Exercise

Stimulation of the mind increases the number and strength of connections between the brain cells, strengthens the brain cells you have, and even increases the number of brain cells slightly. Examples of mental exercises that are particularly effective include solving puzzles, learning something new, reading challenging material, playing board games, playing a musical instrument, and dancing.

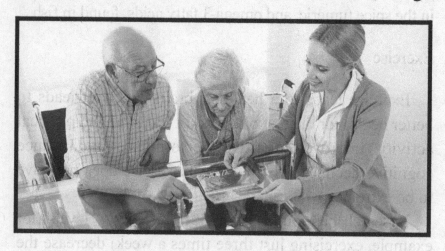

Protect Your Head

Head injury is associated with increased risk for dementia. Protect your head with helmets during sports, wear seat belts, and avoid sports and situations that involve repeated injury to the head.

Socialize

Older people who engage in regular social activities show less cognitive decline. One reason for this effect is that social activities promote new connections between brain cells.

If you are concerned that you might have dementia...

Some forgetfulness is a normal part of aging, but people who forget or misplace things often may begin to worry that they have Alzheimer's disease/dementia. If you are wondering if you should be evaluated for dementia, here are some signs to watch out for:

Do you forget things like people's names or things that you have done recently?

Do you have difficulty cooking, cleaning, or doing other everyday tasks?

Do you misplace things like keys or glasses more often than normal?

If you are concerned, the best thing to do is to talk to your primary care doctor. There are some simple tests that the doctor can perform in the office, and he/she can refer you to a memory clinic or other specialist if needed. There are things that can be done to help reduce the symptoms, so be sure to seek help early. Read our Diagnosing Dementia page to find out how doctors determine if someone has dementia.

If you have been recently diagnosed with dementia...

Getting a diagnosis of Alzheimer's disease or another dementia can be overwhelming. After diagnosis, you will probably feel a range of emotions; fear or anger are very common initial reactions. You might also feel guilty knowing that you will eventually need to rely on family and friends to care for you.

Or, you may even feel relief because a diagnosis of dementia confirms that something was wrong and you aren't just "crazy." All of these reactions are completely normal.

If you are feeling some of these emotions, you may find it helpful to talk with a friend, doctor, or therapist. Or, you may enjoy keeping a journal of your thoughts. Writing in a journal or diary may also help you keep track of things that need to be done, or tasks that you have already completed.

You might also want to consider joining a support group or an online community. It may be difficult to get motivated, but it is important during the earlier stages of dementia to spend time with family and friends doing activities that you all enjoy. You might also want to read about what you can do to slow down the progression of dementia.

What Should I Expect Down the Road?

Every form of dementia has a somewhat unique set of symptoms, and each person experiences the symptoms a little differently. There are some symptoms that are primarily associated with certain dementias. It might be years before you develop these symptoms, or they might be mild at first but then gradually get worse.

Alzheimer's Disease

- Difficulty learning new things.
- Difficulty finding words and forgetting names of people and objects.
- Becoming confused about where you are.

Vascular Dementia

- Difficulty solving problems.
- Difficulty walking, or problems accomplishing other physical tasks.
- Sudden onset and a "stepwise" progression, meaning that symptoms may suddenly get worse, unlike Alzheimer's which has a slower, more gradual progression.

Lewy Body Dementia

If you have Lewy Body Dementia (LBD), you may notice some symptoms that resemble Parkinson's Disease:

- Moving slowly.
- Standing very stiffly.

You may also notice some symptoms that resemble Alzheimer's Disease

- Problems making new memories.

However, there are some symptoms that are unique to LBD:

- Hallucinations.
- Becoming more active at night, and acting out dreams.
- Symptoms improving or worsening over short amounts of time.

Frontotemporal Dementia

- Losing interest in everything.
- Needing to be constantly active.
- Losing the ability to make safe decisions.
- Difficulty understanding and recognizing words or faces. Or, trouble finding the right word to use.

The memory loss and other cognitive changes characteristic of Alzheimer's disease and most other forms of dementia can't be reversed. But there are some proven ways to delay further decline, at least over the short term.

The Rush Memory and Aging Project is a large ongoing longitudinal study looking at common chronic conditions of aging with an emphasis on decline in cognitive and motor function and risk of Alzheimer's. A continuously updated list of scholarly publications featuring research conducted by study investigators can be found on the Rush University Medical Center website.

Mental Activity

A growing body of research indicates that stimulating the brain has the power to slow the progress of Alzheimer's, particularly in the early stages. More-frequent cognitive activity across the life span is linked to slower cognitive decline later in life, according to the Rush Memory and Aging Project.

What you can do:

Encourage the person in your care to participate in activities she finds pleasurable, especially those that engage the mind: reading, writing, playing the piano, working crosswords or puzzle books, playing games such as chess, or even learning a language. Present her with fresh materials or plenty of opportunities.

Local senior centers and adult daycare programs are more than just a way to "pass the time." They excel at providing stimulating activities, including group storytelling, music, art, and games.

Some research suggests that activities are especially protective when they involve interacting with others. Healthy people who are socially active tend to have fewer memory problems than those who are more reclusive.

Arrange for help around the home, if possible, but avoid relieving her of all her customary responsibilities. Participating in daily chores can be a form of mental workout, too.

The catch with mental stimulation:

It's important that someone with dementia finds the activity pleasurable. If she finds studying Spanish or learning to use a computer frustrating because of existing cognitive declines, don't push it.

Also avoid formal mental "exercises" or memory drills. They may stress her, causing symptoms to worsen.

Too much social activity can also be stressful. Outings are best when low-key (small dinners as opposed to, say, big parties) and when they last under two hours.

Daily Life Modifications

Simplifying the living environment and providing the tools to assist her existing memory can help her maintain independence longer. This has the benefit of reducing stress and slowing further decline.

What you can do:

Find ways to minimize any tasks she may worry about. For example, you could arrange electronic bill paying, hire a lawn service, enlist a young neighbor to handle her laundry, or cancel subscriptions to magazines she never reads.

Help her keep her home free of piled-up newspapers, old mail, and other clutter. Look into electronic reminder systems, note-keeping systems, or commercially available tools that can help to prop up a faulty memory.

The catch with daily life modifications:

Be sure to make changes gradually. Too many abrupt changes — removing all the clutter from a messy home in one sweep, for example — can be disorienting and stressful to someone with Alzheimer's or other forms of dementia and hasten her decline rather than slowing it.

Routine and Familiarity

The stimulation of fresh ideas can have positive effects, but too much change in her life can be confusing and disorienting. Familiarity is very important to someone with Alzheimer's disease or other form of dementia.

The stress of having to cope with sudden or significant change can make symptoms worse. (Note: Stress doesn't cause Alzheimer's, but it has been shown to worsen symptoms in those already affected.)

What you can do:

Try to give her day a regular rhythm, with meals, sleep, outings, and bathing happening at about the same times each day. Schedule all doctors' appointments at roughly the same time if you can, such as first thing in the morning or right after lunch. It's not unlike the way a new parent organizes the day around a baby's sleep-wake cycle.

The catch with routines:

A good routine is one that's healthy to begin with. Examples of negative routines worth trying to change: If she's staying awake later and later and rising later, or if she's dropped all former social connections and rarely sees anyone.

Vitamins and Herbs

Scientists are investigating several different dietary additions for people with dementia. Two of the most promising areas:

Antioxidants

A clinical trial showed that vitamin E helps slow down mental impairment in people with Alzheimer's. Vitamin E is an antioxidant, which helps protect cells against damage. It's now being researched in conjunction with B vitamins.

A large 2005 study found that healthy people who consumed more than 400 micrograms (the recommended daily amount for adults) of folate, a B vitamin that occurs naturally in many foods, cut their risk of developing Alzheimer's in half. This slowing of cognitive decline is being looked at to see if it's also true once decline has started.

Ginkgo biloba

This herb, traditionally used in Chinese medicine, comes from the dried leaves of the gingko (maidenhair) tree. It's sometimes called the "memory herb," after findings that it appears to help slow down cognitive decline for some people in the early stages of Alzheimer's disease.

To date, research studies making this claim have been criticized, however, and a randomized clinical trial sponsored in part by the National Institute on Aging and the National Center for Complementary and Alternative Medicine found the herb to be ineffective in reducing the development of dementia and Alzheimer's disease in older people.

What you can do:

Encourage the person in your care to inform her primary-care doctor about any supplements and herbs she's been taking, and their dosages, and do so yourself if she doesn't. Bring the bottle, so the doctor can see exactly what's being taken. Too much vitamin E, for example, can cause gastrointestinal problems and other side effects, and can be fatal to people with heart disease.

In general, the best way to get important vitamins and minerals is to consume them from their natural food sources. One study found that Alzheimer's patients who most closely followed a Mediterranean-style diet (high in vegetables, legumes, cereals, fruit, fish, poultry, dairy, and monounstaturated fats — and low in saturated fats), lived an average of 1.3 years longer than those who consumed a Western diet (higher in saturated fats and meats, lower in vegetables).

Try to make sure that she's eating a diet low in saturated fats and rich in vitamins E, C, and B. Older people's diets often lack fresh fruits and vegetables (such as citrus, berries, and leafy green vegetables), legumes (beans), whole-wheat or fortified bread, and nuts and seeds.

Take a close look at her eating habits. People with memory problems often slack off on cooking because even the familiar steps, as well as managing cutlery, become too challenging.

The catch with vitamins and herbs:

The one thing scientists agree on concerning memory loss and supplements is that more research is needed. No single "magic bullet" has been found to stop memory decline in its tracks, and no supplements should be taken by people with Alzheimer's or other forms of dementia without medical supervision.

Medications

Five FDA-approved drugs are used to delay the symptoms of Alzheimer's disease or prevent them from becoming worse for a limited time.

What you can do:

Talk to your loved one's doctor about which drugs might be appropriate. For mild to moderate Alzheimer's, cholinesterase inhibitors — such as Aricept (donepezil), Exelon (rivastigmine), and Razadyne (galantamine), formerly called Reminyl — may be prescribed.

These medications help keep the enzyme acetylcholinesterase from reducing acetylcholine, which affects mental capabilities and muscle control. The drug Cognex (tacrine hydrochloride) was prescribed in the past, but is no longer recommended.

For moderate to severe stages, the drug Namenda (memantine) is also used. This drug is an N-methyl-D-aspartate (NMDA) receptor antagonist, which regulates glutamate (a chemical messenger in the brain that's associated with learning and memory).

The catch with medications:

Not every drug works for all patients. And each involves possible side effects and interactions with other drugs the person in your care may be taking. Talk to her doctor about whether any of these medications is a good fit.

How Vitamin B Slows Alzheimer's Progression:

The effects of diet on Alzheimer's Disease has been well researched and proved over and over again. Now, a new study conducted by Oxford's Nuffield Department of Clinical Neurosciences has found that vitamin B plays an important role in the slowing of Alzheimer's Disease. Vitamin B is found in foods like shellfish, liver, fish, some cereals, red meat, cheese, eggs, and dairy.

How Vitamin B Slows Alzheimer's

What is Vitamin B?

Vitamin B was once thought to be a single vitamin but we now know that it is actually a group of substances that are not chemically related but are often found in the same foods.

This group of water-soluble vitamins plays an important role in cell metabolism and includes the vitamins thiamin, riboflavin, niacin, pantothenic acid, pyridoxine, biotin, folic acid, and cobalamins. The main role of vitamin B is to keep cells healthy and prevent anemia.

The Role of Vitamin B & Alzheimer's Disease

A new study from Oxford's Nuffield Department of Clinical Neurosciences has found another benefit of vitamin B. The study included over 150 seniors who had mild cognitive impairment and were at high risk of developing Alzheimer's Disease or dementia.

Some participants received a vitamin B supplement while others received a placebo pill. Researchers observed the amount of grey matter in the brain over two years through MRI technology in both groups. Grey matter in the brain shrinks with the development of cognitive decline, dementia, and Alzheimer's Disease.

While both groups had grey matter shrink over the two-year span, those taking the vitamin B supplement had less grey matter shrinkage than the placebo group.

The study abstract concluded that, "Our results show that B-vitamin supplementation can slow the atrophy of specific brain regions that are a key component of the AD process and that are associated with cognitive decline."

Eating more vitamin B

Vitamin B is found in a variety of foods and not getting enough vitamin B can have dangerous side effects. Eat more of these foods to ensure you are getting the vitamin B you need to stay healthy:

- Fish
- Poultry
- Meat
- Eggs
- Dairy
- Beans
- Peas
- Leafy green vegetables

Some cereals and breads have added vitamin B.

What are your favorite foods to eat that are rich in vitamin B? Has a vitamin B supplement helped to slow dementia in your loved one?

If you, any family members or friends are diagnosed with Alzheimer's Disease which is a brain disease that slowly but surely devastates mental, emotional and finally even physical functionality. Alzheimer's is the leading cause of dementia in people over the age of 65 and affects over 300,000 people. Most of the conventional neurologists will in all likelihood offer you just two treatments.

The prescription drug donepezil (Aricept) is one that increases the levels of acetylcholineinthe in the body; it is a brain chemical responsible for memory. Vitamin E is the other. It is an antioxidant that slows the destruction of our brain cells.

Now even though neurologists used to believe that treating Alzheimer's Disease with vitamin E was of no use, recent studies show that the nutrients in vitamin E are effective in the slowing of the progression of the disease.

Although these two treatments are very helpful, there is much more you can do for Alzheimer's. There are natural treatments that can also potentially slow down the progression of this disease and possibly even prevent its later stages.

Your brain is an organ just like your heart. Just as there are treatments plus ways to slow the progression of heart disease, like dietary changes, nutritional supplements, stress reduction and exercise, there are also ways to slow the progression of Alzheimer's.

If diagnosed with Alzheimer's, you must accept the fact that it is a serious health issue and take proper care of yourself and your body. Don't just take a few pills each day, prescription drugs or not. Focus on the fact that your brain has a disease and it is progressive so commit time to tackle the problem and if nothing else, let's slow the disease.

All the natural home remedies here should be part of your regime to fight this but because of the seriousness of Alzheimer's, do so only with the approval and supervision of your physician with a full range of tests and treatments needed to diagnose Alzheimer's.

HUPERZINE A: Slow Memory Loss without Side Effects.

This is the active ingredient in Chinese herb club moss, which has a similar effect on the brain to the drug donepezil, but without the cost or the nasty side effects which include gastrointestinal upsets and liver damage. The purified ingredients of club moss blocks the breakdown of acetylcholine, the neurotransmitter important for memory.

PHOSPHATIDYLSERINE: Boost Mental Capacity.

Phosphatidylserine helps regenerate the outside layer of neurons, reversing the chronological age of these cells by as much as 12 years and improving the mental capacity in Alzheimer's patients. 300 milligrams per day divided into three doses with meals is recommended.

VITAMIN E: Regenerate Brain Cells.

Vitamin E helps shield neurons from free radicals, the unstable molecules that can damage your cells. It can also help regenerate the areas on neurons where neurotransmitters, the chemicals that relay the messages from one neuron to another, enter.

For Alzheimer's patients, it is recommended that 2000 international units a day of the d-alpha tocopherol form of the nutrient is the most effective.

Also important is keeping active as regular physical exercise can help an Alzheimer's patient form new brain cells. Even a daily walk, if possible, is helpful and if necessary, have a friend relative or caregiver go with you even if it is just around the back yard.

CHAPTER TWELVE

Providing Successful Dementia Therapy

Aromatherapy in dementia

In a consensus statement published by the British Association for Psychopharmacology, the use of aromatherapy as an adjunct to the pharmacological treatment of dementia is supported by one of the highest levels of scientific evidence - evidence from randomized controlled trials.

A number of recent, controlled studies have shown that aromatherapy (the therapeutic use of pure plant essential oils) can be useful in the management of patients with dementia: lavender (Lavandula angustifolia or Lavandula officinalis) and lemon balm (Melissa officinalis) are two essential oils of particular interest in this area.

The results of these studies are interesting as their findings cannot be dismissed as merely resulting from the placebo effect of a pleasant-smelling fragrance. Most people with severe dementia will have lost any meaningful sense of smell because of the early loss of olfactory neurons.

Indeed, the pharmacological mechanism by which aromatherapy produces its effects is not thought to involve any perception of odour. Instead, the active compounds are thought to enter the body (by absorption through the lungs or olfactory mucosa) and be delivered to the brain via the bloodstream, where they elicit direct actions.

Aromatherapy studies in patients with dementia

A large number of small, uncontrolled case studies have demonstrated the efficacy of inhaled and/or topical lavender oil in this setting. In summary, these studies have shown lavender oil to improve sleep patterns, and to improve behaviour.

Although only a few controlled studies have investigated the potential use of aromatherapy for the management of behavioural problems in people with dementia, the results have been positive. A single-blind, case-controlled study investigated the effects of lavender essential oil on disordered behaviour in patients with severe dementia.

Patients (n=21) were randomized to receive massage only, lavender essential oil administered as massage or lavender oil administered via inhalation plus conversation. Of the three patient groups, those receiving the essential oil in a massage showed a significantly greater reduction in the frequency of excessive motor behaviour.

In a small (n=15) double-blind, placebo-controlled, crossover trial in patients with severe dementia on an NHS care ward, 2% lavender oil was administered in an aroma diffuser on the ward for a 2-hour period, alternated with placebo (water) every other day, for a total of ten treatment sessions.

According to the group median Pittsburgh Agitation Scale score, treatment with lavender aromatherapy reduced agitated behaviour significantly (p=0.016) in patients with severe dementia compared with placebo, with 60% of patients experiencing some benefit. No adverse effects were reported and compliance with therapy was 100%.

In a crossover study, 56 elderly patients with moderate to severe dementia were massaged with a cream containing a blend of four essential oils (lavender, sweet marjoram, patchouli and vetiver), or cream alone five times a day for 8 weeks.

Behavioural problems and resistance to care were significantly lower in patients who received the cream containing the essential oils compared with those who received the cream alone.

Although most people with severe dementia have little sense of smell, the researchers assessing the study may be able to identify the essential oil being tested, which could compromise a double-blind study.

This problem can be overcome in various ways, such as using observational measures as the primary outcomes of the study, supplying researchers with masks infused with fragrance or nose clips to wear when assessing participants, infusing the environment with control fragrances and masking the aroma of the essential oil with air fresheners.

In addition, as large placebo responses have been observed in many studies investigating the treatment of behavioural or psychiatric symptoms in people with dementia, it is important in studies investigating the effects of essential oils that the control and aromatherapy interventions involve similar amounts of time and touch with each participant.

The researchers concluded that although there is much case-based evidence suggesting the efficacy of aromatherapy in improving sleep, agitated behaviours and resistance to care in dementia, there is a marked lack of adequately sized, placebo-controlled, randomized studies in this area.

Although one placebo-controlled study has shown evidence that aromatherapy may be effective as an adjunct to existing therapy in the management of patients with dementia, this study had a number of methodological flaws.

Essential oils are administered by massage in various 'carriers' (e.g. skin creams, massage oils), and therefore involve the 'additional therapy' of physical contact with carers. Clearly, this additional therapy needs to be minimised or controlled before direct inferences can be made about the effects of aromatherapy alone.

If it is accepted that there are active neurochemical differences between essential oils, then research should investigate not only the oils from different genuses, but should also compare those from related species (e.g. Lavandula angustifolia and Lavandula officinalis).

Properly conducted, well-designed, randomized, controlled trials are required before firm conclusions regarding the efficacy and safety of essential oils can be drawn.

Dementia therapy is a way for a family to provide dementia activities to promote and maintain independence and mental function for as long as possible. Being proactive and starting treatment early and aggressively is important to the person diagnosed with dementia and the family members that provide care for that individual.

Many family members think that dementia therapy is just taking medications. They do not realize that there are many aspects to this condition and medications are just one tiny part of dementia treatment. Before I go any further in explaining the keys to providing successful treatment at home, it is important that you understand that there are many causes and types of dementia.

Once you have a diagnosis, it is important to learn as much about the specific treatment, as dementia therapy has many different approaches. Early intervention and aggressive treatment is often delayed by family members or the patient themselves. This delay can cause serious setbacks or unnecessary progression of the loss of mental functioning.

There are many different types of dementia. The parts of the brain affected, the disease process progression expected (slow versus aggressive), and the prognosis will determine how to plan for future care needs. So, key number one is to learn as much as you can about the specific dementia type and how the different parts of the brain will be affected.

This will help the family and the patient to identify potential future care needs. When a person inflicted with dementia is diagnosed early, they can work with family members and health care providers to make their wishes for future care needs known.

Safety is the second important key to providing dementia treatment at home. Falls are a major concern as we age. Some with dementia will have problems with wandering. Addressing safety issues in the home is important. Making simple changes to the environment may be your first step. Taking measures to keep an individual safe in the home and keep them from wandering outside the home may take a little more expertise.

A certified aging in place specialist can make recommendations to changes to the home environment. An occupational therapist that deals with dementia can make suggestions for things related to the activities of daily living.

Proper nutrition and regular daily exercise is the third key to successful treatment that begins at home. Research studies show that physical exercise is as important as brain fitness exercises to improving mental functioning. Exercise helps the brain create new connections and this, in turn, improves the connections between brain cells.

There are many different approaches and therapies to maintain mental function for as long as possible. It is important that the care givers learn how to focus on the positive abilities of the person with dementia.

The care giver should realize that when the individual they are caring for loses an ability to do something, they will not regain that function back with progressive dementias.

Cognitive therapy, therapies that stimulate sensory perception and learning to communicate with the individual at their present level of functioning are the fourth key. Providing successful care at home means developing a routine with dementia activities.

On any given day that routine may be disrupted. The individual may no longer remember how to do something they did just a day ago. The person providing the care for the individual with dementia with the proper approach can avoid many negative behaviors that can arise out of frustration with care.

The fifth key is the importance of learning behavior modification techniques. One thing for certain is, there will be moments where the person you are caring for will become frustrated, angry or even aggressive. It is important to be prepared to know how to act when negative behaviors are exhibited.

Successful dementia therapy begins at home. Start early, develop short and long term goals and develop an ongoing care plan that changes as the needs of the individual change.

CHAPTER THIRTEEN

Keep Dementia at Bay

MOST CAREGIVERS CAN tell you that Alzheimer's disease and related dementias affect more than just memory loss. The disease often also leads to behavior changes, from simple repetitive behaviors and lost interest in past hobbies to extreme agitation and violence.

Through strategic steps, caregivers can develop a plan to minimize problem behaviors and increase the quality of life for seniors with Alzheimer's disease and dementia.

The first step is to identify the problem behaviors that are occurring and determine the highest priority.

Upon identifying the problem, gather as much information about it as possible. There may be multiple interacting factors contributing to the problem.

Consider the what, when, where, who, how and why.

- • What is actually happening?
- - Describe the behavior(s) observed.

- • What is happening in the environment?
- - Note the noise level (TV, radio, alarms, people) and lighting (bright, dim)? What gestures and facial expressions do you see on the person and those around them? Do you detect any odors?

- • When does it happen?
- - Note the time that the behavior takes place. Is it after a regular event (bathing, mealtime, visiting hours, shift change, taking medication)? Does it happen on certain days or at a certain time of the day?

- • Where does it happen?
- - Does it happen in a specific place? Is it a crowded area? Does location seem to make any difference?

- • Who is around when the problem occurs?
- - Does anyone look or sound flustered, angry, frightened, or threatening? Does anyone remind the person of someone he or she may be prejudiced against? Does it happen when the nurse or caregiver is fatigued or preoccupied? Does it only happen when they're not around? Remember to include yourself.

- • How did the behavior start?
- - There is always a cause for the behavior, though it might be difficult to determine. Try to figure out what happened

just before the behavior. Did it start suddenly or slowly build over time? Were there any clues that it was going to happen?

- Why is it a problem?

- Always ask "why" a behavior is a problem and whose problem it is. If it doesn't make the person with dementia uncomfortable and isn't unsafe, it might not actually be an issue.

Look at the information you collect and create a plan of action. Remember that the person with Alzheimer's disease or dementia cannot change, so it is up to the caregiver to make changes to alter the difficult behaviors.

Keep in mind that behaviors accompanying Alzheimer's disease or dementia are often not normal, so the solutions may also seem farfetched. Write your plan down so it can be reviewed and altered, as needed.

Next, put the plan into action. All members of the care-team should be aware of the plan so it can be carried out consistently. An activity does not need to be a formal exercise, it can be as small as taking a few minutes to look at a magazine or sing a song.

Review the results. Did the behavior change? If so, was it for the better or worse? Did some behavior improve while some got worse? There may be more than one behavior going on at a time. Record what worked and share the information with other caregivers.

Continue re-evaluating your plan and make changes as necessary. The behavior of people with Alzheimer's disease and dementia changes constantly. A plan of action should be reviewed frequently to see if it needs altering - something that worked yesterday may not necessarily work again today.

A flexible approach is essential in dealing with constant changing behavior. People with Alzheimer's or dementia will have "good" days and "bad" days, just as we all do.

Here are several guidelines to keep in mind when addressing behavior problems when caring for seniors with Alzheimer's disease and dementia:

- Review communication techniques - listening to what a person with Alzheimer's disease or dementia is saying, both verbally and non-verbally, is very important for managing behavior problems. Caregivers should also be aware of their own verbal and nonverbal communication.
- Plan ahead for situations that could result in problem behaviors.
- Trying to argue or reason with someone who has Alzheimer's disease or dementia will only result in frustration for the caregiver and the person with dementia - it's not possible to win an argument with a person who has Alzheimer's disease or dementia.

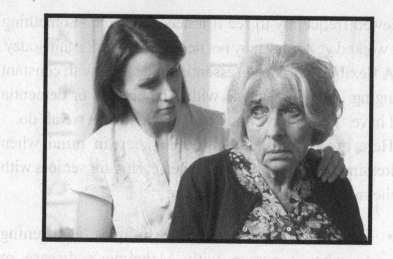

- Keep a routine - changes in routine are upsetting to people with Alzheimer's disease and can cause problem behaviors.
- Positive reinforcements, such as food, smiles, gentle touch, personal attention, and praise are much more effective than negative reactions.

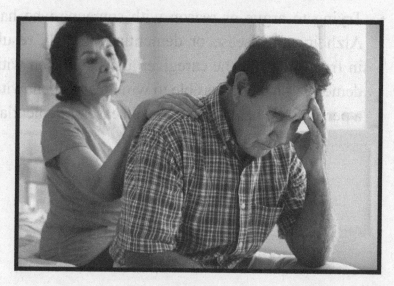

- Allow a person with Alzheimer's disease or dementia some sense of control. Preserving dignity is important, even to someone who is very confused.
- Maintain a calm manner, even when confronted with threatening behaviors. This can defuse a very tense situation and help a person become less fearful.
- Keep things simple. Complex situations cause frustration and escalate behavior issues for people with Alzheimer's disease and dementia.
- Remember that behavioral problems result from the disease. Don't take things that a person with dementia says and does personally. It is the disease speaking.
- Try to keep a sense of humor, even in difficult situations. Humor helps with coping with the frustration of caring for people with Alzheimer's disease and dementia.

It is also important for caregivers to care for themselves. Caregivers should practice ways to reduce stress when they become frustrated and angry.

If a caregiver becomes frustrated or angry, it is best to find someone else to handle the problem so the caregiver can leave the area. A frustrated and angry caregiver will only intensify problem behaviors.

Working with a home care company can be a huge help to overwhelmed family caregivers who need a bit of respite to care for themselves and avoid burning out.

CHAPTER FOURTEEN

Prediction of Disease Spread with MRI Scans

A NEW WAY of analyzing MRI scans looks like it might be able to predict the spread of dementia within the elderly.

The technique works by giving a clearer image of just where the brain degeneration is going and identifies possible pathways that the degeneration might take. This method also shows the promise of being able to predict the rate of progression of the disease.

This image looks at whole brain topography and tries to identify where the expanding Alzheimer's disease or other dementia illnesses is most likely to spread to. The MRI's whole brain topography identifies where the different portions of the brain are connected and pinpoints the pathways where thoughts and actions are processed.

The study looked at 14 healthy brain models and had a virtual "disease" play its course throughout the model human brains. The hypothesis is that Alzheimer's spreads in a similar pattern to prion diseases and researchers used the patterns that these diseases take when accounting for their model computer simulations.

Prions are mis-folded proteins and when they progress throughout the brain, it is thought that they cause other proteins within the brain to mis-fold as well. This in turn can affect someone's brain in an adverse manner.

Protein deposits are often cited as a cause of Alzheimer's disease, so the fact that these two different types of diseases follow a similar structure and pattern is not that surprising.

After the model brains were infected with the disease and it had run its course, the researchers then looked at the actual brains of 18 individuals suffering from advanced dementia and 18 patients suffering from frontotemporal dementia. The results of both the ill brains and the computer models very closely matched each other.

It's thought that with this new technological aspect of analyzing Alzheimer's and other dementia illnesses that precautions might be made someday to help protect memory and other cognitive functioning. This is a long way off, but it is at least one step closer to helping to effectively treat these diseases.

The implications here are big. Now that we can predict where and how fast dementia will spread, we can better know which areas of cognition will be affected and in what order.

This is a big step forward for the treatment of these diseases. And while it's not a cure, it is very likely going to be useful in the future search for one.

Alzheimer's disease is brutal and can affect other family members as they are saddened and frustrated by their loved one's decline in cognitive abilities and functioning. Knowing what to expect isn't necessarily a replacement for a healthy loved one, but the foreknowledge might be of a little help in the grieving and coping processes.

CHAPTER FIFTEEN

How Brain Building Can Help Delay Alzheimer's and Dementia

BRAIN BUILDING GAMES are quickly becoming a popular pastime and mental workout for many people; especially individuals who are concerned that their mental clarity may begin to diminish as they grow older.

In the past, most people were aware of the fact that they needed to give their body a workout in order to maintain good physical health; however, it was only recently that the benefit and importance of brain building games became widely recognized.

As concern regarding Alzheimer's becomes more pronounced, more and more people are turning to brain building games to help keep their brains in tip top shape.

Today's brain building games are much more involved than simple crossword puzzles or even Sodoku puzzles. Research points to the fact that a variety of challenging mental activities are the best for ensuring the brain remains fit as well as producing the all important neurons that stimulate mental clarity.

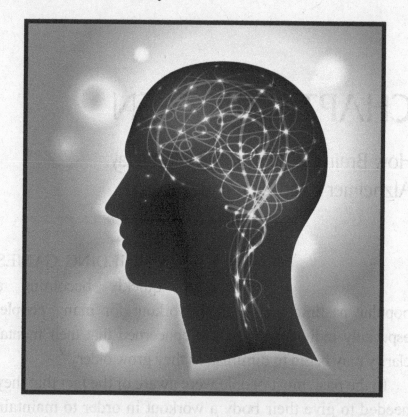

The research is based on the fact that individuals who are able to maintain an adequate level of active brain cells are able to regenerate new brain cells and stave off the reduced mental capacity that frequently plagues many older individuals. Therefore, the real key here is prevention and that means keeping the mind active. Brain building games are an excellent way to do that.

When exploring brain building activities, it is important to recognize the value of variety. An overall good fitness program includes different activities such as strength training and aerobic training; both aimed at ensuring the cardio system is kept in good shape.

The same thing is true with keeping the brain in shape. The whole idea is to make sure you are using different parts of the brain to benefit from improved overall function. Examples of different areas which may be exercised with brain building games include motor skills, language, memory, visual skills and problem solving.

Of course, none of this is to say that Sodoku puzzles or crossword puzzles do no have merit; however, to attain real benefits, it is important to make sure that you participate in a wide variety of activities that involve many different areas of the brain.

In response to the overwhelming interest in building and improving brain function, many manufacturers have come out with a variety of different puzzles, games and activities; all of which are aimed at helping consumers improve their mental clarity.

In fact, such brain building games and exercise equipment has become highly sought after, especially by individuals who are nearing retirement age or who have already retired.

In addition to a wide number of brain building games that are available online, there are also many hand held electric brain building games which make it possible for consumers to take their mental exercises with them. Such games and exercises include memory and reasoning exercises as well as word hunts and games.

Ideally, performing such tasks and exercises at least once per week will provide individuals with the reserve their brains need in the event they do develop dementia or Alzheimer's. While Alzheimer's cannot really be prevented, building a strong mental reserve can delay the onset of the disease.

Living on your own, you miss the input and support of others, whether a spouse, partner or a child that will not leave home. The little things you do daily probably do not amount to much and the daily routine becomes ensconced in your life. Without the presence of others within the home environment, it is easy to miss a slow degradation of mental processes.

The research done today allows us to live healthier lives and making informed choices to live longer. A brief memory loss here and there goes unnoticed, admittedly, and most of us have this at some points in our lives, but it is the slow losses mounting into an inability to cope that become an increasing problem in the world today.

In an effort to delay the onset of dementia or Alzheimer's disease, the authorities suggest that a closer look at diets, foods, and lifestyles is worth considering. We accept that as we age we get the occasional loss of memory. Take the car keys, for example, I think we have all wandered around looking for them.

In order to work correctly, the brain requires certain foods, minerals, antioxidants and vitamins. More attention is paid today into the activity of certain foods providing the research into the dementia diseases. People living longer are facing an increased likelihood of suffering these diseases.

Recent research shows a diet with certain ingredients assists in the improvement of memory processes.

Omega 3 is a well-known fish ingredient linked to reducing the risks of dementia or at the very least, improving brain health. Not only is it useful for brain health, it is also beneficial for improving cardiovascular health. Eating more fish or omega 3 capsules ensures a consistent supply of this nutrient is available for the body's use.

Folates are another major ingredient that should be included in a healthy diet. If your memory is failing you suggests that you are likely to be low in folates. Eat asparagus, broccoli, cranberry juice, liver and up your intake of folate.

Planning to be a mother suggests women take folate tablets prior to becoming pregnant, and certainly over the first trimester of pregnancy. Give the foetus brain the best possible start in life, one that will carry over into later life.

Choline in the form of eggs, soybeans and nuts has a marked effect on boosting memory in older people. Tests have shown that ensuring the addition of these to the older person's diet improves minor memory lapses. Fluids like water must be included every day to maintain the hydration of the body. Dehydration affects the overall performance of the brain and the body's cells.

Anti-oxidants and their effects on our bodies is more widely researched today. The capacity of the body to produce antioxidants to reduce the damage of free radicals is a limited one. Foods with antioxidants include blueberries, red bush teas, and cranberries, even turmeric, are useful in limiting the damage.

Homocysteine is a natural substance found in our blood. High levels of this may increase the likelihood of Alzheimers, or dementia. B vitamins in a diet, particularly B6 and B12, reduce the high levels of homocysteine and may delay the onset of dementia in some cases. A diet consisting of fruit, nuts, vegetables, fish, and chicken is associated with reducing the risks of dementia and Alzheimer's.

While diets are extremely helpful with Alzheimer's and dementia diseases, there are physical means of assisting the protection the foods provide. Keeping your brain busy and interested in life is another means of delaying or avoiding dementia. Brain games using word games or Sudoko can challenge the brain and the cells therein.

Travel and social occasions are part of most people lives, but pay attention to them as we age. It is easy to slip into a mind numbing routine and lose interest in social activities. Without the constant interaction of our families or our social network buddies, the stimulation of the brain cells starts to drop, starting the slow decline in those with a genetic disposition to the dementia diseases.

CHAPTER SIXTEEN

How to Become a Successful Alzheimer's Disease Caregiver

ALZHEIMER'S DISEASE is a progressive disease where the condition worsens over time. As more parts of the brain are being damaged, the symptoms of Alzheimer's disease become more severe. Patients experience frustration and grief as they struggle with gradual loss of function and fading memory.

Their family members grieve as well, as they observe their loved ones losing their abilities, personality and function. Anger, confusion, sadness and depression are common reactions in families experiencing anticipatory grief.

Being an Alzheimer's caregiver takes energy and courage. As the patient's mental abilities decreases, the caregiver's responsibility increases. Thus, the caring for a patient with Alzheimer's disease could become increasingly difficult and stressful over time.

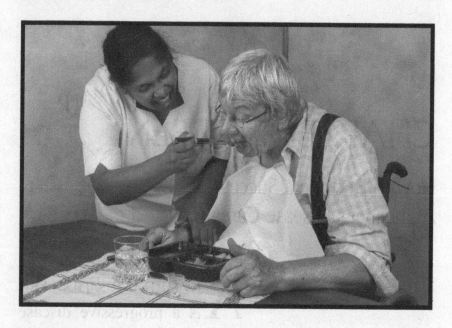

Many Alzheimer's disease caregivers experience intense stress as they struggle to understand the patient's behavioural changes and determine what interventions will work for the problems that arise each day. This stressful task can have a detrimental effect on the caregiver's emotional, social and physical well-being.

One possible way that the caregiver could reduce the stress of caregiving and cope with the task more effectively is to develop skills in caregiving.

As Alzheimer's disease progresses and the behavior of the patient becomes more complex, caregivers need to understand the patient's changing behaviors and learn techniques to manage the behavioural difficulties.

Thus, it is particularly important that the caregiver acquire knowledge about the Alzheimer's disease and its progression, skills and strategies for managing the challenges, and information on the available resources to turn to when the need arises.

This is even more essential if the caregiver is new to the task. If a new caregiver has totally no knowledge of Alzheimer's disease and is greatly lacking in coping skills, the task of caregiving is even more difficult.

Along the way, as the caregiver encounters more and more unexpected new challenges, the caregiver will definitely feel overwhelmed by these problems. The stress experienced by the caregiver would certainly be greater and could result in a detrimental effect on the caregiver's well-being, which in turn could result in an adverse impact on the patient's situation.

It is also important to note that every patient deserves the highest standard of care possible and an equipped caregiver is more able to provide the high standard of care required for the patient.

At times, although an elderly person with severe impairment in memory and mental function may need to be communicated with at the primary functioning level of a small child, he or she also needs, and has a right to be respected as an adult.

A trained caregiver would learn the communication skills required to interact with the patient and be more equipped to provide proper care for the patient.

Hence, training is necessary for the caregiver to acquire the appropriate skills needed for the job and enable the caregiver to provide the standard of care required. The patient will benefit from the quality of care provided.

Thus, the importance of developing skills in caregiving should not be overlooked. It would certainly help the caregiver to cope with the task and reduce the stress of caregiving. At the same time, the caregiver will be able to provide the standard of care required and the patient will benefit from it.

Furthermore, if caregivers find that their approaches are effective, they will gain confidence and increased satisfaction doing the task. In this way, hopefully, caregivers would end up finding meaning and purpose in the difficult task of caregiving instead of finding the task a daunting one.

GET YOURSELF AS A SUITABLE CARER AT HOME FOR YOUR LOVED ONE

There is nothing simple about living with a terminally ill loved one at home, or living with this on your own. There are many big decisions that you'll be facing and none of them are going to be easy to make.

You probably already realize that each new day brings new challenges. Most of these decisions will need to carefully thought out to ensure that they are the right ones for everyone.

Many family members at home want to be the one to take care of their loved one. This desire isn't always the best course of action to offer the best possible care. The reality is, you need to work and live your life. This type of care will hinder your career, social life and overall future.

The care that you will be able to offer might be limited. It's understandable you want to do whatever you can for your loved person, but there are better options for optimal care.

One option is to place your loved one into a hospice. This isn't to say it is going to be an easy choice, but it might be the best. Weighing out your options will help you to find the best type of care for your loved one as well as the entire family.

There are many advantages to hospice care and there will be some disadvantages as well. It is important that you understand what they all are. Talking with the hospice directly will help to give you all of the necessary information. You should contact someone to discuss the type of care that your loved one will receive while in their care.

A hospice is filled with many professionals including physicians, nurses, social services and bereavement staff to guide you through the unfortunate time. Supportive care such as this helps not only your loved one, but also the entire family.

The first steps you will need to take is making a phone call to a hospice and learning more about what they have to offer. You will uncover that the guidance and direction they offer is everything that you had hoped for. Reading more about hospice care online is also a great starting point. It helps you to ask the right questions when you speak to a doctor on staff.

These next few weeks are going to be hectic while you begin your planning process. You'll find that there are many loose ends that will need to be tended to such as preparations for power of attorney, updating life insurance policies, making copies of important documents, and so much more. It is easy to get overwhelmed.

THINGS TO REMEMBER AS A DEMENTIA CAREGIVER

The sad reality of dementia is that the dementia patient gradually starts to forget. At first it seems like stress or fatigue may be the cause, but as the forgetfulness increases and other symptoms become evident, the dementia caregiver may become nervous about some of the important information that could be lost in their loved one's memory.

While caring for a dementia patient, it is easy to get caught up in the day to day tasks that can claim so much time. While preparing meals, making a safe environment, and tending to health care needs are important and very necessary, there are other aspects of the dementia patient's care that must be taken care of also.

Schedule and plans

We all lead busy lives. We have hobbies and interests and clubs and work obligations and friends and family. A dementia patient's schedule doesn't suddenly empty because they become forgetful. If anything, it may become even fuller because they may double (or even triple) book themselves without realizing it.

Knowing your loved one's schedule and plans will help you to help them to organize their time and commitments.

Knowing where they will be at any given time has the added benefit of helping to keep them safe. If they don't show up for an appointment or if they are late returning home, you will have valuable information to aid in a search for them.

Filing system

As their memory declines, the dementia patient will require more and more help with financial, legal, personal, and professional paperwork. Knowing where to find pertinent information will be extremely helpful for the dementia caregiver.

Even if a dementia patient has kept meticulous records throughout their adult life, the nature of dementia may cause them to become slack in putting papers where they belong or may even cause them to rearrange files.

Understanding how to use their filing system and helping them to keep it updated can save the dementia caregiver much time and stress.

Financial information

While it may feel like you are prying into their affairs by asking about their income and their budget, financial mismanagement is one of the earliest signs of dementia problems. At some point, the dementia patient will become unable to handle their own finances.

In the meantime, they will still have bills to pay and possibly even debt that needs to be taken care of. The problem with becoming forgetful is that the dementia patient is likely to forget to pay bills on time or even at all while adding to their expenses of buying things they don't need or giving away money they don't have to give.

As early as possible, the dementia caregiver needs to learn about the financial affairs of their loved one and help the dementia patient to take the necessary legal steps to have someone take control of this area of their lives when it becomes necessary.

Insurance information

As a person ages, their insurance needs change. It may be difficult at this point in a dementia patient's life to increase or add insurance where needed, but it is also possible that they may be over-insured in some areas.

Beyond the financial aspects of insurance bills, there are the available benefits of the coverage they carry. Knowing what is covered and what is not covered, how to make a claim, which doctors they can see or can't see under their plan, whether or not other people are allowed to drive their vehicles, etc. This is all valuable information that can either cost the dementia patient money or save them money.

Work with them to locate and understand all of their insurance policies.

Medical history

A written record of the dementia patient's medical history is critical. Knowing when they have had surgery or been treated for a particular disease can be invaluable in helping a doctor in making decisions about their current and future care.

Help them to compile a list of surgeries and medical treatments, including all prescription medications they have taken or are currently taking. Looking through their files may provide some of this information if they are unable to remember it.

Final wishes

Watching a dementia patient slip away is heartbreaking. Knowing that eventually it will be time to make tough decisions concerning their medical and physical care and ultimately the details of their burial can be daunting.

Have a conversation about these things while the dementia patient can still express their desires. Take notes.

Help them to get the necessary legal documents in place so they will have someone to make these decisions for them when they no longer can.

Contact Information

We interact with a lot of people and businesses in our daily lives. The older we get, the longer the list of friends, family members, and acquaintances becomes. The dementia patient may forget who some of these people are, much less how to contact them.

Help the dementia patient to continue relationships as long as possible and help them to let their friends and family members know about their dementia symptoms. This will help to provide closure for both parties.

Then, keep a record of all of the contact information for these people so that you can contact them if, and when, you need to.

Where valuables are stored

We all misplace things. A dementia patient can misplace many things. They may have intended for years to give a cherished family heirloom to their oldest child, but then the item suddenly disappears never to be located.

Whether they sell these treasured items, hide them very well, throw them in the trash, or give them away to someone else doesn't matter, the item is still gone.

If your loved one has such items, help them to start giving them to their intended recipients now. This will help to avoid hurt feelings as well as help to pare down their belongings in case they need to move to smaller living quarters.

Family recipes

Take the time to cook and bake with your loved one. Not only will you be able to spend precious time with them, but it will also give you a chance to record their "secret" ingredients so you will be able to recreate those wonderful tastes.

Family history

Elderly people are a wealth of information. One thing they are especially good at remembering is family stories. While you may be tired of hearing a dementia patient repeat the same stories over and over again, the information they contain about your family history is priceless.

Record these stories either with a voice recorder or by writing them down. The details of their and your past will be treasured by future generations.

As I mentioned at the beginning of this chapter, just the details of every day life can seem overwhelming to a dementia caregiver. Finding the time and energy to add the additional steps mentioned in this chapter may be overwhelming.

CARING FOR PEOPLE WITH DEMENTIA

Dementia, is a condition that involves a person losing their cognitive abilities. However, this is not the same as the normal levels of cognitive deterioration that are a part of the aging process.

Sometimes, dementia can have a progressive effect due to disease or damage; however it can also stay the same if the sufferer has had an injury to their brain. Most cases of dementia are present in older people, however it can happen prior to aging and this is known as early onset dementia.

In a country that has an aging population, like Britain, the numbers of people suffering from dementia are likely to increase. As such, it is important that people have an understanding of what dementia is, and how people suffering from it can be treated and helped to live with a degree of normality.

World Health Organisation statistics suggested that the worldwide number of sufferers was around 35.6 million in 2010 and is set to rise by around 70% by 2050.

If dementia is diagnosed early on, then steps can be taken in order to make sure that the patient can have an improved quality of life, and some of these steps include dementia aids.

It is important for the patient to be helped to try and retain as much independence as possible, in order to help the patient feel that they are still in control of their lives, and also to ease the pressure on those caring for them.

One way in which life can be made easier for the sufferer and the care giver, is the use of dementia aids and dementia products. These products are designed to stand out to the patient, so that they know what the items are and what they are used for.

A speech by David Cameron emphasised the seriousness of dementia in the UK and outlined how hospitals and other facilities will be made more dementia friendly, to help patients and care givers feel more at home and comfortable.

What Dementia Aids Are Available?

There are a range of dementia aids available that will help those giving care to a dementia patient and patients themselves cope better which include:

Memory boxes - These have become increasingly popular and are designed to keep things that have a meaning to the patient from aspects of their lifetime. This is a way for those caring for them to jog their memory about the past and have things to use as a conversation starter, to help your patient feel at home.

Toileting aids - In order to help your patients have a better ability to retain their independence, aids such as brightly coloured toilets seats can help your patient's remember what needs to take place. Similarly, other aids in the bathroom such as grab rails and other support devices can help those who struggle with manoeuvrability.

Incontinence products - Although the two aren't always related, one side effect of dementia can be incontinence - in order to ease the embarrassment of this as a condition, incontinence products are available which allow the patient to carry on with life as normal as possible, in a dignified manner.

What are the most appropriate dementia aids?

There are no right or wrong options in terms of selecting dementia aids, different patients will have different needs. The most important thing to consider when caring for someone with dementia is to try as much as possible to interact with them as normal, and try to instil a feeling of independence.

By using various dementia aids, the patient can still have a sense of having their personal freedom and this can help reduce the strain on their carers.

CHOOSING ACTIVITIES TO DO WITH THE DEMENTIA PATIENT

As a dementia caregiver, you may get so busy "caring" that you don't take the time to have fun. Participating in activities, whether they are practical or frivolous, can boost your spirits and also boost the spirits of your care recipient. But how do you choose these activities?

Dementia patients are sometimes brushed aside with the thinking that they no longer have the ability to actively pursue any of their former interests or to learn new skills. This is often not the case.

A dementia patient may not have the ability to initiate an activity, a hobby, or a game, but if they are given the proper materials and patient step-by-step instructions, they may not only be able to participate, but also to thoroughly enjoy themselves.

The behavior problems that are common with dementia patients may be lessened if the patient is given the chance to express themselves through art, music, or some other medium. Activities also have the added benefit of burning up energy which may help the dementia patient to sleep better.

Here are some tips for choosing activities to do with a dementia patient

What did your loved one enjoy before they developed dementia symptoms? They will most likely continue to enjoy the same activities. Some hobbies, especially sports or potentially dangerous activities, may need to be modified for the dementia patient to be able to participate, but although they may not be able to safely climb a mountain, they may be able to continue to go on short hikes.

Be creative. Creativity will help you to find ways to modify activities. Consider all the aspects of a particular interest. For example, if your loved one loved to play Sunday afternoon football with his buddies, perhaps he would enjoy watching football on TV with his friends.

Some dementia patients become a little childlike in their actions. Participating in activities that are usually reserved for childhood may be enjoyable for them. Finger painting, playing marbles or jacks, or swinging on a swing set at the park are all great ideas. If possible, do these kinds of activities with a child.

Dementia patients often remember events and experiences from years ago, but can't recall what they had for breakfast an hour ago. Reminiscing about their childhood or their wedding day or their time in the military can be enjoyable for them. Working on scrapbooks or interviewing them about these events are great ideas for activities.

Keep it simple. The more steps it takes to complete a project, the more likely it will be for a dementia patient to become confused. Choose activities with only a few steps and be sure to break down each step as simply as possible when giving instructions.

We all want to feel needed. This is no different for a dementia patient. Every activity they participate in doesn't have to be fun and games. The opportunity to be helpful can be very valuable. Simple chores like folding laundry, pairing socks, tearing lettuce for a salad, scooping cookie dough, and many others can all be done successfully by a dementia patient.

When choosing activities for a dementia patient there are many possibilities. See your loved one as a vibrant, productive member of your family and of society and you will be able to find many things for them to do. Provide a little instruction and watch them enjoy participating in life.

SIMPLE EXERCISES FOR DEMENTIA PATIENTS

Studies have shown that exercise for people with dementia is one way for individuals to cope with this debilitating disease.

In many instances, there has been a tremendous amount of improvement in both cognitive and physical skills in individuals suffering from dementia when a quality exercise program is introduced into the treatment process.

Although the exact link between exercise and the cause of dementia has yet to be defined, the establishment of an exercise program in the daily lifestyle of individuals who have been diagnosed with dementia, individuals with a family history of dementia, or individuals with beginning symptoms of dementia. When it comes to the specific types of exercise for people with dementia, consider the following four tips.

1 - Seasonal exercise for people with dementia

Seasonal exercise is incredibly important when it comes to those individuals with dementia.

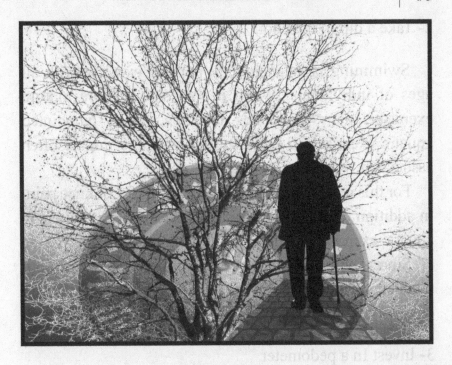

In addition to allowing individuals to alter the exercise plan in an attempt to avoid the routine from becoming stale or tired, these seasonal exercises often allow individuals to enjoy the fresh air of the great outdoors whenever possible. For example, a fantastic seasonal exercise is enjoying a brisk walk in the park.

Depending on your area, you may want to consider altering the time of your daily exercise routine.

The early morning or late evening hours are especially popular for outdoor activities for those especially hot or humid areas of the country. In order for your seasonal exercise to benefit you year-round, consider choosing exercises that can be adapted for the great indoors as well.

2- Take a dip in the pool

Swimming is an incredibly popular exercise with all ages of individuals. When it comes to a more mature exerciser, many physicians have specifically pinpointed aquatic exercises in order to eliminate the impact often associated with exercise.

For this reason, individuals with back, hip, or knee pain, in addition to those individuals with arthritis, often enjoy aquatic exercises for the lack of pain.

Since swimming can be enjoyed year-round in both outdoor and indoor pools, consider joining a specialty group or class in your area that focuses on aquatic exercises.

3- Invest In a pedometer

The amount of steps you take in a given day may be surprising. Doctors suggest that individuals walk anywhere between one-half to one and one-half miles in a given day.

To keep track of just how many steps you are taking, consider investing in a pedometer.

This unique device is simple to use and easy to carry. Even if you are not interested in counting your steps, a pedometer may be one way to allow you to remember to complete your exercises. These small devices are widely available for purchase in your local sporting goods shop or sporting goods section of a larger retail store.

Furthermore, a pedometer is quite inexpensive, and can make an excellent gift for anyone looking to expand his or her exercise program.

4 - Exercise your mind

Especially for individuals with dementia, the most important exercise is the exercise of the mind. Some games are simple and easy, making them perfect for enjoying with all ages.

Many individuals, who have been diagnosed with dementia or who have been experiencing the beginning signs of dementia, often enjoy playing simple games with their children or grandchildren.

While spending quality time with their family, individuals with dementia can work towards stopping and potentially even reversing the impact of the disease.

If you are interested in specific exercises that are appropriate for mental health, consider speaking with your primary health care provider or seek specialist services in a doctor that deals specifically with the many diseases of dementia.

CHAPTER SEVENTEEN

A Guide to Homecare

THERE ARE MANY reasons why families should start considering the option of elderly home care for their senior loved ones. The growth of elderly home care services and care home senior day care centers these days assures us that growing old is now becoming a simpler process for the elderly.

Many people do not consider the option of home care for their older adults because they feel that it might be too expensive. This is not the case, as care at home can be more economical than a care home - not to mention the benefit it has for your loved ones and the family as a whole.

There are a lot of elderly home care services that can offer a wide range of care services, including: respite care, live-in care, specialist care for dementia, strokes,

Parkinsons and end of life care. Good care agencies will be dignity champion supporters, working hard to ensure that each individual client is treated with dignity and respect.

Their top priority is to ensure that the individual is safeguarded from harm, comfortable and is provided with an environment that helps them maintain their independence, respects their choice and individuality as well as keeping them safe.

These home care services are uniquely tailored for you, and if you are not sure what service and care best suits you or your loved one, then don't worry because the Care Manager will meet with you to assess and discuss your needs and requirements.

There are some care givers that provide night time services, dementia and Alzheimer patient services, end of life services, live in services etc. With so many services being provided by these various home care services, there will be a good solution for you and your loved ones to receive the best possible care to meet their needs.

Most of the good home care service providers employ trained professionals. These professionals are highly trained, they will have been CRB checked, trained in safer manual handling of people, trained in personal care, followed the essential standards of care and received a thorough induction by their company.

Some people may be entitled to financial support from the government. An individual can be means tested and assessed for their needs requirement by a local social worker. Please contact your local county council for more information, especially if you have concern for the safety and safeguarding of an elderly or vulnerable adult in your area.

Before you consider any kind of care provider for your relative, it is imperative that you do your own research to find the best. You can talk to friends and family about these services.

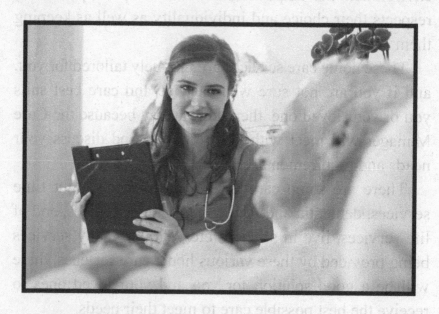

People might be able to give you some names about good home care providers near you.

Once you have a list of names, you will need to review these care givers thoroughly. Make sure that trained individuals are working for the company. You will also need to go and speak to these companies in person and ask any relevant questions that you may have in your mind.

You will need to thoroughly outline the needs of the patient/older adult to the companies. Pay attention to the specifications so that there is no negligence on your part or theirs.

Once you've made up your mind about who to hire, and you've provided them with all the information that they will need, you should stay around for a while to see how they are taking care of the person in question. Make random checks to inspect their services until you are satisfied completely that you have a good service provider working for your relative.

DEMENTIA SAFETY IN YOUR LOVED ONE'S HOME

Individuals with memory loss and confusion are at risk of harming themselves because their judgment is impaired, so dementia safety precautions are vital. They may not remember how to use a band aid, go outside without wearing a winter coat or may eat food that has grown moldy Individuals in the early stages of Alzheimer's disease or other types of dementia begin to require supervision in order to be safe. At the same time, certain home adaptations can increase peace of mind for caregivers.

Doing a Home Safety Assessment

Occupational therapists are trained to perform home safety assessments for dementia safety with special attention to factors that might contribute to falls, consuming toxins and injuries from sharp objects or fire.

Caregivers should also think about adapting a loved one's home, much in the same way parents with young children child proof. Here are some adaptations that I made when my mother was living alone in a Senior Housing building before relocating to an assisted living residence with memory impairment services:

• Removed old newspapers, grocery receipts, magazines, bags and other clutter.
• Removed candles, matches, sharp knives and other dangerous tools.
• Removed toxins including bleach, which has a container that looks like a gallon of milk and cough syrup which smells like candy.
• Disabled the microwave and electric stove.
• Provided a shower seat (the apartment already had grab bars).
• Added night lights with sensors that turned them on at night.
• Regularly checked food for freshness.
• Removed small rugs.

Creating a Home Environment that Promotes Independence

The removal of clutter not only increases dementia safety and decreases the chance of fire, but will make it easier for the person to find important items such as keys, eyeglasses and wallet.

Fill the refrigerator with only ready to eat foods such as hard boiled eggs, tuna fish sandwiches and cut up vegetables. Technology creates an undue frustration for individuals with memory loss. However, here are a few tips that helped my mother:

- Set the television to her favorite station and tape over all buttons except the on/off switch. Highlight that switch with bright orange nail polish.
- Preset number one on the telephone to dial a "helper" friend or relative. Then highlight the number using nail polish and place a sign next to the phone that says "Push number 1 for help."
- Remove all remote controls.
- Buy lamps that go on and off when touched.
- Provide a digital clock that includes the date and day of the week. Digital clocks are easier to interpret than face clocks.

Routines and Visual Cues

Individuals with memory loss have a great deal of difficulty learning new tasks. However, they will probably have greater success continuing familiar routines such as putting dishes in the sink after meals or sequencing steps to get dressed. Caregivers should try to maintain the familiar routines as best as possible.

Sometimes. visual cues such as a note next to the sink that says, "Use soap" may provide the cue needed to perform a routine action. Laying the towel on the sink counter also prompts the person to use it. Setting up the environment with visual reminders will help the person in the early stages of memory loss to remain as independent as possible.

SAFETY PROOFING YOUR HOME FOR ALZHEIMER'S DISEASE

Many caregivers are choosing to have their loved one remain at home rather than placing them in a skilled nursing facility.

This works well when plans are made for the safety of the loved one with Alzheimer's disease and the well-being of the caregiver is considered. Home is familiar, home produces a sense of security, and home means home.

In some ways, planning for the safety of a victim with Alzheimer's is like preparing for the advancing independence of a busy toddler. The distressing thing is that the caregiver often is forced to move in reverse.

While the toddler gains in comprehension of safety issues, the person with Alzheimer's forgets more and more. The familiar becomes the unfamiliar and that is worrisome and dangerous.

Start with the bedroom. Is the bed set at a level where first steps in the morning land gently on the floor rather than in a leap to it? A bed too high needs to be lowered. Later, a safety rail should be installed so that your loved one does not fall out of bed and injure herself.

A bed pushed next to the wall is also advised since now there is just one exit from the bed. A rug with an alarm or a "baby" monitor is wise, especially when the caregiver is sleeping or working in another room. The noise awakens the caregiver before too much activity can ensue.

Dressers and closets serve best when they are cleared of too many objects and clothing choices. Choice can become confusing and so clothes may be tossed and shoeboxes strewn and tripping becomes a danger.

Many times, the loved one with Alzheimer's becomes attached to certain items of clothing - a favorite shirt and comfy pants, for example.

Purchasing several sets that are just alike to make dressing simple while also allowing dirty clothes to be washed because favored clean clothes are at hand. Slipovers with wide necks and pull-up pants with no zippers will make the potential dressing fiascos self-dissolve.

Be sure that hallways and other walkways are clear. Rugs can be baffling. A dark one may look like a hole; a light one may resemble a step; a toe tangle in one can result in a fall. Stair steps also present a danger.

If bedrooms are upstairs, a safety guard should be installed so that an inadvertent late night stroll does not become a rolling disaster. In later stages, the bedroom may need to be moved downstairs as the up and down of steps can become puzzling and fearsome.

Your bathroom needs safety latches on cabinets where any medications or cleaning supplies are stored. Easy on and off faucets are nice so that the victim can remain a bit independent, and so that the caregiver can use fingertips and elbows to assist with washing. Showers and bathtubs appear like menacing traps.

They are loud echo chambers, in many cases, and running water adds to the unclear understanding of what is happening. Often, those with Alzheimer's resist bathing for reasons including the exposed nakedness to cold and other eyes, the frightful step into a deep tub, the plunge into the mystery of water, or the sprinkle of a shower that zaps the face.

A removable showerhead works wonders in both bath and shower. It is gentle and easily adjusted and allows for cleaning in private places without being too invasive. A bathtub bench that slides is handy.

The "showeree" sits on the bench while the "showerer" lifts legs and carefully slides his loved one into the bath. Stepping is avoided plus standing for a long time becomes difficult so the seat serves as a rescue. Showers can be easier to maneuver since the step is small and with your new removable showerhead installed, water flow is set to perfection.

Be sure to purchase soft washrags and towels and shampoo and soap that are no-tear. Having wrestled a loved one into the bath should not be exacerbated with burning eyes and rough rags and wipes.

Meals need to be simple for you, the overworked caregiver, and for the loved one with Alzheimer's as she loses the skills of using knife, fork, and spoon or drinking from a glass. Finger foods are advised, cut into smaller and smaller bites to avoid choking. A cup with a lid and straw work well.

Getting your loved one to eat and drink enough becomes challenging so a handy store of simple food and drink is useful. One-inch squares of peanut butter sandwich are nutritious - just be careful of food allergies. Bananas, sliced peaches or pears, cheese cubes, and other soft food add to a balanced diet.

Milk is source an excellent vitamin, although both my mother and sister who died of Alzheimer's, developed dairy allergies and our "forcing" milk turned into intestinal repercussions. Juice, water, and even some pop add to essential liquid intake.

In the kitchen, stove knobs should not turn easily to "On" (tape may be needed to secure them), refrigerators and oven doors may need latches, cabinets may need safety catches, and high tables and chairs may have to be eschewed for lower seating.

While Mom may still want to cook, know that supervision may be required. Although Dad still wants to wash dishes and put them away, prepare yourself for less-than-clean and overly chipped dinnerware. Patience is the greatest virtue a caregiver can possess.

Now for the living and/or family room. Comfortable seating and a favorite chair make for a homey atmosphere. For many with Alzheimer's disease, hearing may fail so the volume may go up. When blasting television drives you to blasting fury, try to relax.

Often, you can turn the volume down without your loved one noticing and when he turns it back up, leave the room then return to lower it once again. In time, your loved one will not be able to follow the storyline of shows and TV may become a waste and annoyance.

It is then that you'll treasure those irritating days of blasting blabbering as your loved one sinks into the quietness and vast sense of loss of this incurable disease.

Final, for in-home safety, lock the doors. You do not want your loved one strolling the neighborhood alone while you put clothes in the dryer. Be sure that locks are secure and that knobs and latches do not turn, thus releasing the locking mechanism.

Also be sure that you have spare keys hidden outside. It is easy to rush out the door to intercept your loved one as the door crashes closed behind you.

Your wobbly sense of preplanning will stabilize a bit after you have chatted with friends and neighbors about your loved one, your concerns, and the possibility of wandering. You also should contact your local police department to alert them of potential wandering.

I have found that when people know your angst, they step up to support your caregiving in good times as well as during crisis. And when they don't, it seems that there is always an individual in the wings (literally as I call them angels) to reinforce your strength and determination as you care for a loved one with Alzheimer's disease.

CHAPTER EIGHTEEN

Future Dementia Treatments and Cure

A CURE FOR dementia is what most people want and scientists have made great progress in finding one. Here's what you need to know about future treatments - some of which might be just around the corner.

In a nutshell

Dementia is a complex condition with many possible causes, but what many people want to know is, can dementia be cured? Finding a cure is never going to be easy, but recent developments and understanding of how the disease progresses have been encouraging. Researchers now believe an effective treatment – if not a complete cure – could be available within 10 years.

Three reasons to hope

1. In the 1970s, a war was declared on cancer which has had significant effects in developing new and powerful treatments. A similar 'war' was declared on dementia at the 2013 G8 Summit when dementia was finally recognised as one of the most serious medical challenges of the 21st century.

2. More money than ever before is being poured into research. The UK government has pledged to double its annual research funding to £132m by 2025.

3. World experts are coming together to pool funds and resources and share information. As a result, scientists now have a better understanding of the mechanisms involved in the diseases that cause dementia than ever before.

So what could future treatments offer?

Here's a few of the drugs and therapies that are currently being researched and developed in the fight against dementia.

1. Disease Modification Therapies (DMT)

The current drugs available to treat Alzheimer's and dementia tackle the symptoms of the disease, but a new type of medication called Disease Modification Therapies works by tackling the disease itself and could potentially be of far more benefit. These drugs are being hailed as a 'transformative event' in the search for a cure. Watch out for one called Solanezumab which is currently undergoing clinical trials.

2. The diabetes connection

A drug called Liraglutide, currently used to treat type 2 Diabetes, could become the first treatment to reverse the progression of Alzheimer's disease. A £5m study is currently under way in the UK after the drug was shown to reduce the damage caused by dementia when tested on mice. It is thought that the drug could be particularly beneficial to people in the later stages of dementia.

3. Ultrasound *2 yr away*

Canadian researchers have found a way to remove toxic amyloid plaques in brain cells (which have long been associated with Alzheimer's) by using a non- invasive form of ultrasound. Although it hasn't been tested on humans yet - human trials are at least two years away - scientists say this could be a breakthrough which fundamentally changes our understanding of how to treat Alzheimer's.

4. A vaccine

A new vaccine called Betabloc could halt the advance of Alzheimer's and also repair any damage already done. The vaccine works by attacking the amyloid plaques on brain cells. The vaccine doesn't only remove the plaques, it also restores mental function. Clinical trials are already happening.

5. A drug to ease agitation

A new drug called <u>Brexiprazole</u>, which could help to reduce agitation in people with moderate to severe dementia, is doing well in trials. The drug may offer a safer and more effective way to manage behaviour problems than the other anti-psychotic drugs currently on offer, and it could become available within a couple of years.

The future looks bright

Here's what worldwide dementia experts have said recently.

'In my generation, the aspiration is that by 2020 or 2025, we will find a treatment for dementia or at least the commonest cause of dementia which is Alzheimer's disease.'

The future is bright, and there is a lot to be enthusiastic about, but we aren't quite there yet.'

Professor Alistair Burns, NHS director for dementia.

'We now understand much more about the progression of Alzheimer's disease and researchers are finding ways to identify people in the earliest stages where they have the best chance of developing treatments that work.'

Researchers around the world are working to develop effective treatments for dementia, and eventually to find a cure.

Much of this work is focussed on Alzheimer's disease, the most common form of dementia.

There is currently no cure for Alzheimer's disease. Available medications can reduce symptoms and improve quality of life in some people, but they do not stop the progress of the disease.

The potential treatments discussed below are in the early stages of research and are not currently available. However, they are all part of the research effort to find more effective treatments for Alzheimer's disease and ultimately a cure.

Alzheimer's vaccine and Immunotherapy

Researchers have been attempting to develop a vaccine for Alzheimer's disease for almost a decade. The strategy behind the immunotherapy approach is to use the body's own immune system to destroy beta-amyloid plaques.

The first Alzheimer's vaccine was tested in clinical trials in 2001. However, the trial was prematurely halted because six percent of participants developed serious brain inflammation.

However, the vaccination did appear to benefit thinking and memory in some unaffected participants who were monitored after the end of the trial. Researchers have now developed a safer vaccine by using antibodies against a smaller fragment of the beta-amyloid protein, which they hope will avoid the complications of the previous trial.

Another approach to developing a vaccine involves using immunoglobulin, a filtered human blood product containing antibodies. Immunoglobulin was shown to be successful in a very small trial of 8 people with mild

Alzheimer's disease, with most showing improvement on tests of cognitive function after treatment.

Although this trial is very small, it suggests the potential for larger trials of immunoglobulin therapy, which may have safety advantages over other vaccination techniques. Although this initial research is promising, much more research needs to be done before we know whether this approach will work.

Gene therapy

Gene therapy has been promoted as a promising technique for many different conditions. A very small trial of gene therapy for Alzheimer's disease has shown beneficial effects - slowing the progression of the disease by about 50%. In this trial, genetically modified cells were injected directly into the brain.

The cells were modified to produce nerve growth factor, a natural substance that helps brain cells to grow, survive and repair damage. Although the study is very preliminary, it indicates that gene therapy may provide beneficial treatment for Alzheimer's disease in the future.

Targeting beta-amyloid production

Several treatment strategies for Alzheimer's disease rely on targeting the production of beta-amyloid or its accumulation into plaques. One such strategy focuses on trying to inhibit the activity of enzymes which are involved in the production of the beta-amyloid protein.

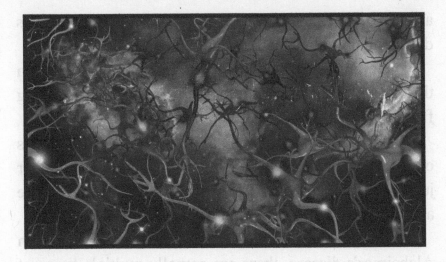

The enzymes beta and gamma secretase act to cut amyloid precursor protein (APP) into several protein fragments, including beta-amyloid. These beta-amyloid fragments then aggregate into plaques. It may be the plaques or the fragments themselves or groups of fragments called oligomers that interfere with and damage nerve cells.

Researchers are trying to develop drugs that inhibit these enzymes in order to reduce the production of plaque forming beta-amyloid. However, as both beta and gamma secretase have many other roles in the body, it has proven difficult to selectively inhibit their effects on APP and beta-amyloid in the brain.

Other strategies to stop beta-amyloid's damaging effects include preventing its accumulation into plaques. Compounds that bind to beta-amyloid and help to clear it from the brain are being trialled.

Zinc and copper are required for beta-amyloid fragments to form oligomers, so other compounds that target zinc and copper to prevent the formation of beta-amyloid oligomers are also being trialled. Vaccinating against beta-amyloid, as discussed above, is another approach under investigation.

There are many new medical treatments for dementia that have proven successful for many individuals suffering from this common medical condition.

It is believed that as many as 10 percent of individuals over the age of 60 suffer from dementia. That number jumps dramatically to 25 percent of individuals over the age of 80.

Although dementia is most commonly associated with Alzheimer's disease, there are actually multiple types of dementia.

Just like any other medical illness, these different types of dementia have different behaviors and symptoms.

At this time, there is no known cure for any type of dementia, but there are options for medical treatment for dementia available that can slow the progression of the disease and improve the overall quality of life for dementia patients.

Latest Treatments

Physicians are currently treating dementia by focusing on the specific effects of the disease.

Often, many of the effects of dementia are irreversible, especially if left untreated. Although there are not any treatments available that can completely reverse these effects of dementia, there are certainly ways to slow down or potentially stop some of the more serious effects of the disease.

Additionally, these medical treatments for dementia strive to find the root cause of the problem. Although dementia can be a specific disease, it can also be a side effect of another disease. Dementia can be caused by something as simple as incorrect medication or an interaction between two different types of medication.

MEDICATIONS FOR DEMENTIA

Acetylcholinesterase Inhibitors

There are certain types of medication that have been used to treat different types of dementia. The most widely publicized type of medication is undoubtedly the family of Acetylcholinesterase inhibitors.

This type of drug has been approved by the Food and Drug Administration and is currently being used as a medical treatment for Alzheimer's Disease in addition to other types of dementia. The brands associated with these inhibitors include Cognex, Aricept, Reminyl, and Exelon.

These drugs work to inhibit the breakdown of acetylcholine, which is a chemical produced by the brain that allows the nerve cells to communicate.

In most forms of dementia, when acetylocholine is broken down and becomes unable to be properly used by the body, the nerves are unable to communicate.

When the nerves are unable to communicate, the mind is unable to clearly process thoughts. Although these medications have shown progress in delaying the slowing this breakdown and delaying the signs of dementia, they are unable to completely stop or reverse the effects.

Furthermore, once a patient begins taking one of these acetylcholinesterase inhibitors, he or she must remain on the medications indefinitely, since the breakdown can become expedited when the medication is stopped.

N-methyl D-aspartate Blockers

Another type of medication typically used for the treatment of dementia is the N-methyl D-aspartate blockers.

These blockers include Namenda, another Food and Drug Administration approved drug that has shown success in treating those individuals with Alzheimer's.

The body naturally produces a chemical known as glutamate, which can be hazardous to the body if produced in too great a quantity. If exposed to great quantities of this chemical, brain cell activity can decrease and nerve cells can die.

Individuals who have certain types of dementia are found to have increased productivity of glutamate, and these medications can better regulate chemical production.

If you or a loved one has been diagnosed with a type of dementia, know that there are options available that can slow the progression of the disease.

Doctors and researchers are continuing to work towards a cure for all types of dementia, so a cure may be right around the corner.

A List Of Common Dementia Medications

Alzheimer's disease (AD) is the most common form of dementia. Other common types include Lewy body dementia, Parkinson's dementia, and vascular dementia.

There is no known cure for any type of dementia, and medications can't prevent the condition or reverse the brain damage it causes. However, various drugs can provide some symptom relief. Read on to learn what these drugs may do to ease dementia symptoms for you or your loved one.

About medications

Types of dementia medications

Several prescription medications are approved by the Food and Drug Administration (FDA) to treat symptoms of dementia caused by AD. These drugs can provide short-term relief of cognitive (thought-related) dementia symptoms, and some can also help slow the progression of AD-related dementia.

While these drugs are approved to treat symptoms of AD, they're not approved to treat symptoms of other types of dementia. However, researchers are exploring off-label uses of these medications for people with non-AD dementias. According to the Alzheimer's Association, research suggests that some AD medications may benefit people with vascular dementias and Parkinson's dementia.

Some of the most commonly prescribed medications used to treat symptoms of AD are cholinesterase inhibitors and memantine.

Cholinesterase inhibitors

Cholinesterase inhibitors work by increasing a chemical in your brain called acetylcholine that aids in memory and judgment. Increasing the amount of acetylcholine in your brain may delay dementia-related symptoms. It may also prevent them from worsening. The more common side effects of cholinesterase inhibitors include nausea, vomiting, diarrhea, and dizziness.

Examples of commonly prescribed cholinesterase inhibitors are:

Donepezil (Aricept)

Donepezil is approved to delay or slow the symptoms of mild, moderate, and severe AD. It may be used off-label to help reduce behavioral symptoms in some people with thought problems following a stroke, Lewy body dementia, and vascular dementia. Donepezil comes as a tablet and a disintegrating tablet.

Galantamine (Razadyne)

Galantamine is approved to prevent or slow the symptoms of mild to moderate AD. It may be used off-label to help provide the same benefit for people with vascular dementia or Lewy body dementia. Galantamine comes as a tablet, extended-release capsule, and an oral solution.

Rivastigmine (Exelon)

Rivastigmine (Exelon) is approved to prevent or slow the symptoms of mild to moderate AD or mild to moderate Parkinson's dementia. It comes as a capsule or patch.

Memantine

Memantine is used mainly to delay increasing cognitive and behavioral symptoms from moderate to severe AD. This effect may allow people with AD to function more normally for a longer time. Memantine may be used off-label to provide the same benefit for people with vascular dementia.

Memantine is not a cholinesterase inhibitor, but it also acts on chemicals in the brain. What's more, memantine is often prescribed in combination with a cholinesterase inhibitor. An example of this combination is Namzaric, a medication that combines extended-release memantine with donepezil.

Memantine comes as a tablet, an extended-release capsule, and an oral solution. Its more common side effects include:

- Headache
- High blood pressure
- Diarrhea
- Constipation
- Dizziness
- Confusion
- Cough
- Infection with the flu

Effectiveness

How effective a dementia drug is varies by drug. For all of these drugs, however, the effectiveness tends to reduce over time.

Takeaway

Talk with your doctor

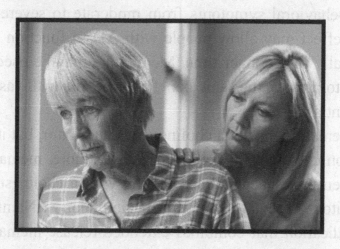

While there is no cure for dementia, several prescription medications can help slow the progression of the cognitive effects and other symptoms that dementia can cause.

If you or a loved one has dementia, talk to your doctor about all of your treatment options. Be sure to ask any questions you have, such as:

What type of dementia is it?

Which medications will you prescribe?

What results should I expect from this medication?

What other treatments are available?

How long should I expect this medication to help?

CONCLUSIONS

I HOPE YOU enjoyed reading this book and have found the information useful. There is much that can be done to help dementia sufferers and I'm certain that you will have found some small nuggets of information that you may have been previously unaware of.

The book was written to primarily help sufferers, family members and carers, so that they do not feel alone and abandoned, feeling that there is nothing that can be done. There is much that can be achieved and improved upon with just some small adjustments to daily routines and living arrangements.

Dementia, as we have seen, is a term for a long-term condition which covers several different types of the disease. It can be a difficult and trying time for the patient and for family members who may have to live with or cope with a loved one who is suffering from it, but as we have also seen, there are many things that can be done to alleviate the condition and make for a more comfortable and happy life.

By keeping things as normal as possible, using interesting activities and mild exercise as a therapy, a sufferer can enjoy some normality and stimulation, even when suffering quite severe effects.

I have also created a website with numerous short videos to help you to easily understand all about Dementia and also to update you without delay any important findings from new research as they happen-ie an up to date information source to continue to support you.

You could reach the website at this address: www.DementiaAdvice.Care

There is also a Facebook Page that will enable you to interact with me and a growing community of more than 5,000 Fans & Followers. The link is: www.Facebook.com/DementiaAdvice

I hope that you and your loved ones can discover your own paths to a better life, with the help of the contents herein.

PART II

FREQUENTLY ASKED QUESTIONS ON DEMENTIA AND ALZHEIMER'S DISEASE

By

Selva Sugunendran

CEng, MIEE, MCMI, CHt, MIMDHA,
MBBNLP, MABNLP

#1 Best Selling Author, Speaker & "Success Through
Wellness" Coach © Information Marketing Business

1. Who may be affected by Alzheimer's disease?

Given that Alzheimer's is a disease that can't be traced to a specific cause, we can only speculate on the combination of factors that make some people more vulnerable and likely to suffer from it. The following are some of the most common factors that need to be considered in order to evaluate the level of risk of an individual in case they are experiencing any mild symptoms, which could be completely unrelated to the condition in many situations.

The age of the patient

According to statistics, there will be about one person out of every 20 individuals over 65 years old who will end up developing the condition. The same statistics show that hardly a single person out of one thousand is ever going to develop the condition before they reach 65 years of age. This means that age is definitely a very important risk factor to consider.

A head-injured patient

Evidence has suggested that people who suffer from serious head injuries due to a strong blow are more likely to develop Alzheimer's. The risk is increased dramatically when the person who suffers from the injury is over 50 years old.

Heredity in some patient's families

This is also a factor that needs to be considered. There seems to be a limited number of people who inherit the disease from their parents, but there are many cases of people dying from Alzheimer's and their children not being affected.

The gender of the patient

Studies are also suggesting that women are more likely to get the disease than men are. The truth is that this is the least relevant of the factors that we have mentioned so far because those studies are still very far from conclusive.

Other probably factors to consider

There seems to be a link between education levels and Alzheimer's, but it's still too early to consider this to be a relevant factor to keep in mind. One thing that we can mention is that evidence is suggesting that people with a higher level of education are less likely to develop this condition than those with lower levels of education. This is known as mounting evidence, but more years are required to come up with a precise statement.

Anyone who is over 65 should be given an Alzheimer's test in case they start experiencing any symptoms just to rule out the condition or to be given proper care in case of a positive diagnosis.

2. Signs & Symptoms of Alzheimer's disease

There are many reasons why people would consider going to the doctor when they feel their mental health is not optimal. The truth is that conditions such as Alzheimer's are not always going to be diagnosed if a person is forgetful or feeling disoriented at times, but there are some key signs and symptoms that people who are starting to develop Alzheimer's will generally experience. We are going to go over them so you can have a better idea of what to look for if someone you know is experiencing these symptoms.

Memory loss

This is going to be the initial stage of the condition is most cases. Memory loss can happen due to a large number of things, but frequent problems remembering things, and having to use reminders for things you used to remember on your own are usually signs of a problem.

Planning and problem solving

Simple problems that require the use of logic or mathematics might become challenging all of a sudden. If the problem happens once and it doesn't continue to happen, it will probably be an isolated incident due to being tired or many other factors, but a persistent situation with solving simple problems should be worth checking.

Forgetting how to get certain tasks done

If a person has specific daily tasks at home or enjoys playing a specific board game or card game, they will probably have no problems getting those daily tasks done or playing those games efficiently. If a person is developing this condition, they will have trouble getting those tasks done with the same level of ease as they once did. This would be a good time for an Alzheimer's test to be conducted in order to rule it out or properly diagnose it on a patient.

Being confused about the time or the location

Some people will start to feel like they have a very hard job keeping track of time. They will feel like a day already passed and they will get confused with dates. They might also start to feel forgetful about something as simple as knowing where they are headed when they start walking.

Having problems speaking and writing

When a person starts to have problems finding the right words to say during a conversation, or they feel like it's hard for them to write what they are thinking, they might also be experiencing early signs of Alzheimer's.

3. Understanding signs and symptoms of Alzheimer's disease

Once an individual starts to show signs of mental abilities being lost and difficulty remembering things, this can cause serious concern in the person experiencing those symptoms as well as those around them. The symptoms are noticed by everyone who comes in contact with the person and this means that they will rarely let them go unnoticed or try to hide them because they cannot control when they will show those signs.

It's essential to seek medical attention and get a proper evaluation as early as possible in order to begin proper treatment. This is going to be extremely important because it will give people the time to adjust to the situation and take action. It's very important to understand the signs and symptoms that are often experienced when a person is going through the early stages of Alzheimer's disease.

The mild initial symptoms

The mild symptoms include forgetfulness and having a hard time remembering where you left your car keys and your sunglasses. This is often accompanied by having a harder time expressing thoughts with words and mood changes that happen for no apparent reason. This first stage is usually not going to be too much of a concern until the symptoms worsen and the person seems to be forgetting things quite frequently.

The moderate symptoms

Once Alzheimer's starts to cover more brain tissue, it will start to show moderate symptoms that can become extremely problematic for people. This includes memory loss that makes them forget how to get to places that they have visited frequently and difficulty carrying out tasks as simple as putting on clothes. At this stage, people might even have a hard time recognizing family and friends and it's quite apparent that they are no longer able to function as entirely independent individuals.

The most severe symptoms and stage of Alzheimer's

At this point, all of the symptoms that we have mentioned earlier become even more severe and the person starts to experience problems with the functions of their body. This means they will have a hard time swallowing food and keeping their balance. The progression takes about two years from the beginning stages of the severe symptoms until the person is unable to move efficiently and needs to be in bed all day long.

The progression of each stage will depend on the kind of treatment that is given to each person as well as their age and their general health.

4. What actually happens to the brain over time when Alzheimer's disease progresses

There are many mysteries that surround the reasons why some people get Alzheimer's disease and why most people don't, but the condition is more common than most people imagine. Once it starts, it will start to attack the brain and deteriorate the mental health of the patient.

Being the most common form of dementia, this condition will progress to a fatal outcome even with proper treatment. The search for a cure or at least for a way to stop the progress of Alzheimer's is constant, but for now all we can do is give proper care to those who suffer from it.

According to research, Alzheimer's is caused by the abnormal buildup of plaques that get between the nerve cells in our brain. This creates a chain reaction that slowly destroys brain cells until the patient is unable to do anything on their own. The body will start to shut down slowly, but the progression is steady and impossible to stop with current medical treatments that are available.

The progression of the condition can begin even 20 years prior to symptoms that would prompt someone to seek medical attention for a proper diagnosis. Unfortunately, there is still no way to detect the early stages of the condition.

Once the mild and moderate stages begin, the plaques and the tangles will start to develop in areas of the brain that allow us to use our brains for thinking, planning and memory. That is the moment when people start forgetting things day by day and they feel confused and mildly disoriented. Once this happens, the personal and professional life of the patient will start to be affected and this stage can last as little as two years, but it could also take up to a decade to develop into severe Alzheimer's stages.

The late stages of the condition are terrible for the relatives of the patient because they will become strangers to the person suffering from the condition. They will no longer be able to take care of themselves properly and they won't even know how to get to the bathroom of their own home.

Once this stage sets in, the condition can last for up to 5 years on average before serious health complications set in and the patient needs to be hospitalized while being given proper care until their organs start to shut down completely.

5. Communicating with your doctor about your Alzheimer's disease

There is no question that being diagnosed with this condition is not an easy thing to experience. You will need to maintain a good line of communication with your doctor in order to ensure the best and most optimal treatments during the progression if the disease. Learning how to deal with this with a team effort mentality between you, your doctor and your family is the best way to approach this debilitating condition.

This is the main reason why anyone who is suffering from Alzheimer's should consider proper communication with their doctor while also consider taking other important steps to ensure maximum support. The lack of proper interactions between patients and doctors is going to have a very serious impact in the way that the condition is experienced and also in how long it can be kept from advancing to stages that will make the patient completely dependent on others.

We know that it can be stressful to even consider going to a doctor due to issues with memory loss and disorientation, but the sooner this stage is over with, the easier it is for a doctor to give the kind of treatment that will give the patient results they can trust. Remember that the earlier the diagnosis, the easier it is to plan ahead in every aspect of your life and in the prevention of an aggressive deterioration of your mental abilities. Some people with Alzheimer's are able to live relatively functional lives for well over a decade.

There is also the fact that medical advances are finally showing substantial results that might lead to a cure or at least a stop in the progression of the disease. This is going to make it a lot easier for people to handle their condition and maintain a good level of social interaction during the early and mid-stages of Alzheimer's, while also ensuring comfort during later stages.

Remember that doctor are there to help you move forward in life and to give you the kind of results that will help you live your life as normally as possible given the situation. There are plenty of treatments available right now to help people with Alzheimer's live their lives without serious concerns for a long period of time and this is the reason why you need to keep your communication with your doctor as open as possible.

6. Diagnosing Alzheimer's disease

A series of evaluations of the symptoms the patient is experiencing will be conducted by a doctor and this is the most basic Alzheimer's test that leads to further testing. The first thing that the doctor is going to do is evaluate the earliest signs of the disease. This means looking for episodes of memory loss and impairment e.g. difficulty concentrating and finding it hard to locate certain places that the patient once knew how to find easily.

Other evaluations include the process of checking for language problems and changes in mood that come for no apparent reason and are new to the patient. Distance distortion and not being able to drive properly are also common early signs that doctors will look for when evaluating and diagnosing Alzheimer's.

Another factor to determine the kind of testing needed from that point on is the age of the patient. Most people under 65 years of age are likely to be suffering from other not so serious conditions if they show these symptoms. Very few and rare cases involve people in their late 50's and anyone younger than that is extremely rare. The doctor is also going to evaluate your medical history to see if the patient has ever sustained any head injuries and if they have any other conditions that could contribute to those symptoms.

Interviews with people close to the patient are also going to take place in order to see the perspective of those around them. This is very important because the patient might not see things and remember them the same way that they do. Neuropsychological tests will always be part of the process too. Once those are done, a regular series of clinical exams will be taken in order to rule out any deficiencies and thyroid disorder, which can often be confused with the early signs of dementia.

In conclusion, there is no such thing as an Alzheimer's test in the sense that there are a series of tests that need to be conducted in order to reach a diagnosis. There is no single test that would help determine the situation so that a solid diagnosis could be provided. There are also many other conditions that need to be ruled out and this could make the process even longer. The results will then be used to conclude if the condition is indeed Alzheimer's in order to give the patient proper care for their condition.

7. Preparing for the future during progression of Alzheimer's disease

Alzheimer's is a condition that affects a large number of people all over the world and the need for proper attention, diagnosis and treatment is huge. This is not a condition that a person should experience on their own without any assistance. There will come a time when the individual who is suffering from ALZ is not going to be able to function independently and this is going to be extremely difficult to handle.

Being able to prepare for the future while the disease is still manageable and you have full mental capacity is going to be very important.

Contacting the official Alzheimer's disease organization in your area is going to be very important. The evaluation of each patient with this condition helps with the research for a cure. This does not involve taking part in any kind of experimental drug treatments, but it helps contribute important data that compares all kinds of factors that are very valuable to the medical community.

Once you have done this, you should make sure that you have a doctor that is able to take proper care of your needs. You might choose to continue treatment with the doctor that gives you the diagnosis of your condition, or you can decide to get someone else to see through your treatment in every stage of the condition.

You should also look for a counselor or psychologist because they will help you handle the situation and all of the emotional ups and downs that you will experience when you have Alzheimer's. This is very important and extremely useful because it will give you the chance to find comfort in their professional advice.

Get your personal life in order

While it's hard to even consider this to be an option, we need to act fast and get our life in order when it comes to 3 basic affairs. Our finances, our legal responsibilities and delegations and our medical care expenses. Once you are able to take care of those aspects of your life, you are going to have the required peace of mind to carry on with the journey of experiencing the stages of Alzheimer's without any other worries in your mind.

It's also important to handle those aspects of your life in the early stages of the condition because you might not be able to have the mental capacity to do this at later stages.

8. The future outlook for Alzheimer's patients

There are many conditions and serious illnesses that we are fighting hard to eradicate. Cancer is one of the leading concerns worldwide, but Alzheimer's is definitely another huge problem and the way in which the person starts to slowly deteriorate and fade away is without a doubt something that no one wants to have to experience. The patient suffers in the beginning stages of the condition due to the progression of the limited mental skills and abilities, but then at the later stages of the disease, the condition greatly affects both the patient and those around them.

Aducanumab

This is an antibody that seems to be one of the most promising in stopping the progression of the condition, but there are a total of five DFA approved drugs that are specifically meant for Alzheimer's treatment and they seem to be helping people with temporary boosts in memory and thinking in general. The biggest hurdle with Alzheimer's research is the lack of federal funding for proper research, but there is also the fact that volunteers for clinical trials are not lining up to be used as test subjects.

It makes sense that people with this condition want to be cured, but they are also afraid of being subjected to clinical trials that could have serious side effects on their already weakened bodies and minds. This is one of the reasons why it has been so hard to be able to test the drugs properly and to go back to the drawing board based on results.

The amount of research that is done on this subject is going to be related to the kind of support that is given to the research. Many drugs are being developed that could help stop and even cure the condition, but this is not going to be easy and there is a lot of ground to cover. The only way that the research will be done with a more frantic pace is to raise more awareness about this illness and this is going to allow more chances for funding and donations to be given to the cause.

Alzheimer's is a very peculiar condition because of how it slowly robs the person of their independence and their ability to take proper care of themselves. Finding a cure for it needs to be in our list of priorities if we want results during all of Alzheimer's stages.

9. Preventing Alzheimer's disease

There are many mysteries that surround Alzheimer's disease and being able to prevent the condition is still not entirely possible. With that said, there are some important things that you can do in order to help keep your brain in top condition and this will reduce your chances of getting the disease. We are going to give you some important tips that you can implement in your daily activities to help you decrease the chances of developing Alzheimer's disease.

Your diet is very important

If you eat a lot of junk food and you don't consume nutritious foods that have all the vitamins and minerals your body needs, your immune system will be weaker and this is going to unleash a large number of health issues that could also contribute to suffering from Alzheimer's disease when you reach a certain age.

Eating more fruits and vegetables is going to be very important because your body needs proper nutrition instead of artificially flavored junk food or prepackaged TV meals that fill your stomach with chemicals and make you feel full, but your body is getting very little in terms of nutrients.

It's also important for you to increase the intake of Omega-3 fatty acids because the docosahexaenoic acid that is found in lean meats such as salmon and mackerel is known to lower rates of Alzheimer's. Taking supplements is also going to help and folic acid is one of the most useful and beneficial supplements for your body.

Exercise and meditate

People underestimate the value of exercise combined with meditation. The modern world is very hectic and even senior citizens are part of this fast-paced digital era now. We have gone from counting days, to counting hours just to get things done and even people who are retired are stressed and anxious because their children and grandchildren are always stressed and anxious.

Taking things easy and learning to live life without overcomplicating everything is going to be a great way to keep your body and your mind healthy. Stress is known for having serious effects on our physical health. Our bodies don't work at optimal levels when we are stressed and this lowers our defenses and hurts our immune system. If your immune system is compromised for long periods of time, you will get sick often and serious conditions can develop from this. Many of them contribute to the possibility of Alzheimer's in the future.

10. Understanding Vascular Dementia

There are many causes for dementia. Vascular dementia is caused by a lack of proper blood flow to the brain and a large number of seniors are suffering from this condition all over the world. Just like all types of dementia, this type is gradual and it will start to affect the patient over the years. This particular dementia is the one that can be slowed down the most and people are able to live with it for over a decade in most cases.

There are many symptoms that have been linked to vascular dementia. One of the most common is that people are going to feel as if it has become harder for them to think fast and it seems like they are having a hard time organizing their lives and planning things out. Those symptoms are usually going to involve disorientation and confusion in many situations too and this is usually going to make the person feel concerned enough to visit a doctor for a diagnosis.

Another symptom will include difficulty keeping balance and walking. The truth is that all of these symptoms could be caused by many other conditions, but the important thing to keep in mind is that the combination of all of these symptoms will often lead to the diagnosis of some form of dementia. Not always, but quite often and it's even more likely that a form of dementia is involved if the person is over 60 years-old.

There are several tests that need to be conducted to determine if the person is suffering from dementia. Some of them include the proper assessment of their mental abilities with a series of psychological tests. There will also be a blood tests involved in order to find out if a person is feeling experiencing any kind of blood pressure problem. This can lead to the diagnosis of vascular dementias after MRI and CT scans have also been conducted to see if there is any damage done to the brain in any areas.

There are several treatments that can help a person live with the condition for much longer. Proper diets, weight loss, avoiding consumption of alcohol and tobacco and lowering cholesterol are all going to be extremely helpful factors that will help a person slow down the symptoms and the progression of the disease in a way that is considerably effective.

11. Dementia with Lewy bodies

There are different types of dementia and this is one of the most common that can be diagnosed in people all over the world. The definition of dementia is given to all kinds of brain issues and gradual changes that damage functions slowly but steadily and the symptoms for each type of dementia are different.

The symptoms for this disease are hard to notice at first and they are known to affect all kinds of aspects of a person's life very gradually. This starts by making the person feel like they have trouble understanding things and even thinking about things they once had no problems analyzing.

These symptoms will gradually get worse and the concerns of the patient will become quite apparent. This is why reaching out to a doctor is important. It is worth noting that these symptoms could be due to a large number of issues unrelated to Lewy bodies dementia.

There will be times when the person is going to feel very alert and then they will be confused and sleepy with a lethargic feeling. All of these states will change through the day randomly and they will make the person feel like there is something different about their mood and behavior. This is usually the most common reason why men and women end up being checked and eventually diagnosed with dementia.

The tests that are given to a person to determine if they have Lewy bodies dementia are not specific and a large number of different tests are needed in order to come up with a proper diagnosis. There are brain scans that are often going to be seen as ideal for this diagnosis. The MRI and CT scans are amongst them and they will provide some signs and evidence that can lead to the diagnosis.

The treatments that can be given to people who suffer from Lewy bodies dementia are quite varied. None of these treatments will provide a cure for the condition, but they will help lower the severity of the symptoms until the condition reaches its most severe stages.

People who suffer from this particular dementia are known to survive for 5 to 14 years but some have been able to survive for much longer. It all depends on the kind of care that is given to these people and how they are able to handle and manage the condition.

12. Understanding Frontotemporal Dementia

Out of all of the types of dementia that a person can suffer from, the frontotemporal condition is the one that can strike at the youngest age on average. There are people as young as 45 years-old who are suffering from this condition and it has been known to rarely affect people who are even younger. While most dementia cases of any kind are diagnosed at 65 or older, this type of dementia does have the highest rates of younger people who have been diagnosed with the condition.

This kind of dementia is like any other in the sense that it's also going to start developing slowly and it can take over a decade for the symptoms to reach critical stages. People will experience several symptoms in the early stages and they will eventually start to feel concerned and get initial tests done.

This includes behavioral changes that can seem to be selfish and very impulsive. There are also situations in which a person will experience extreme lack of motivation and difficulty handling social interactions when they once had no problem with them.

The person who is affected with frontotemporal dementia might also start to speak slower and they could feel like getting words out in the proper order could be difficult. This is often very frustrating and it contributes to the mood changes. Being easily distracted and having a hard time organizing and planning things will also be an alarm that something is not right.

There are also going to be memory issues but these are not as common in the early stages of the condition and they are more likely to be experienced after many years in the advanced stages of this particular dementia. A doctor will usually determine the stage of the condition after conducting a series of tests that are going to let the individual find out how they are feeling.

An assessment of the current mental abilities of the individual will be conducted with a series of tests and questions. Blood tests will also be conducted in order to be able to rule out any other conditions that might be causing these symptoms. The MRI, PET and CT scans can be a good idea in order to see what parts of the brain are being affected by the condition and in some cases spinal fluid might be removed to find out if the patient has Alzheimer's.

13. Dementia is a progressive disease

Dementia progression is one of the most difficult things to witness for people who have relatives with this condition. It's a slow disease that takes a long time to affect the brain functions and it has very specific stages that need to be tracked carefully in order to provide the right kind of care to the patient.

Dementia is not always the reason why people are forgetful and they lose things easily. Some older people and even young people experience something called Mild Cognitive Impairment or MCI. This is not necessarily going to develop into Alzheimer's disease, but most cases of Alzheimer's are first diagnosed as MCI and then progress to the disease.

The stages of dementia

Mild dementia is considered to be the first of all dementia stages and people will start showing signs of it with short-term memory loss and misplacing objects often or having trouble expressing themselves. This could last a few years and in some people, it starts with a very mild case that can often be confused with MCI.

Moderate dementia will set in when the person is experiencing disorientation and might even feel like they don't know how to get to a location they already knew. Changes in sleep patterns are also common and personality changes can be noticed at this point as well. This is a stage of dementia that still allow the person to have full motor function, but the mental capacity issues start to be quite apparent.

The severe stages of dementia will start when people completely lose their ability to communicate with others and they will be unable to walk, sit, hold their own head up and even swallow. Then, the patient is not going to be able to control their bladder or bowel functions either and this leads to fatal complications.

Final thoughts

It's hard to say how long it takes for people to see this progression, but it can be years for the most serious symptoms to develop, but it can also start to advance fast depending on each person and their general health. It has been proven that a stress-free environment helps patients with dementia maintain a level of awareness and mental capacity for longer periods of time than those who are constantly stressed due to improper care. This is the reason why customized care plans for every patient with dementia are so relevant.

14. Getting dementia help and advice in the UK

Being able to get the right kind of help and advice when it comes to dementia is going to be extremely important. Thousands of people are diagnosed with many forms of dementia in the UK each year and being able to find the right kind of guidance and advice is going to be essential. This is the reason why the Alzheimer's Society network has been created and you can reach them through www.alzheimers.org.uk in order to find out as much as you want about the problem.

The best thing about this particular organization is that they have a national dementia helpline for people who need advice on what to do. This is also meant to serve as proper guidance in case a person is experiencing symptoms and need to know where to go and what do to next.

There is also a huge community of people who share their experiences and connect with others. The best thing about this is that it provides a perfect support group of people who are going through the exact same thing. This kind of online community really helps those who feel alone and depressed because they will be able to find a large number of people who are also suffering from this condition.

There are many features that are also very attractive. People can volunteer to help those suffering from dementia and there is a support network that is constantly growing to provide the best possible service to anyone who requests help. Training is also provided to anyone who wants to learn how to take proper care of people who are suffering from dementia. This means that they will be given training that is going to help them deal with every stage of the mental deterioration that people with dementia experience.

This is definitely the kind of online platform that deserve to be shared with everyone you know. There is plenty of information available in the website and the community grows day by day. The support system and the encouragement for funding and volunteering is definitely to be considered more than enough to involve people in the process.

Be sure to let everyone know about this great and helpful website that is going to give a large number of people the hope and support they are looking for when dealing with this condition as patients or relatives of a patient.

15. Guidelines for advanced stages of dementia

There are many different factors to consider when a person is suffering from a stage of severe dementia and the kind of approach that is given to the care of a person at that stage is going to have a serious impact on the quality of life that the patient can expect to have. Knowing when the patient could be given medication for chronic conditions and understanding the risks and side effects of each of those medications is essential. This will allow the caregiver and the family of the patient to decide on which course of action to take in order to see the best possible results.

Some healthcare institutions and independent caregivers choose to use a holistic approach to alleviating some issues related to dementia, but those who are at a chronic stage of the disease are more likely to see no substantial comfort derived from this kind of alternative medicine.

The need for 24/7 nursing care is going to be determined by the inability that the patient has when it comes to taking care of their most basic needs. Not being able to feed themselves or not being able to use the bathroom without assistance are clear indicators that this person needs medical attention all day long and it should be seen as a priority to provide nursing care.

The use of antibiotics to take care of certain issues related to advanced stages of dementia is also going to be an important step in the treatment of the condition. Once an individual reaches the final stages of the condition, the need for proper treatment is going to be of paramount importance to alleviate the patient during those final stages of the disease.

Advanced dementia is to be considered a terminal condition and it needs to be treated as such. All of the care and treatment needs of a patient who is terminally ill are going to follow the same protocol regardless of the condition that is causing the terminal stage to begin to take place for any patient.

The substitute decision marker needs to be aware of the many decisions that need to be made at this stage in case the patient hasn't been able to leave all personal and financial matters resolved. The legal issues related to dementia patients should be solved as early as possible with the person still able to make decisions on their own when it comes to legal procedures.

16. How Dementia Progresses and the Stages of the Mental Decline

There are many factors that need to be taken into consideration when the stages of dementia are determined and a time lapse can be provided. The truth is that all we have are average expectancies, but each person is going to be able to handle the condition with a varied degree of resistance to the mental deterioration. This is going to depend on how strong the person is and how good their physical and mental shape has been up to the point of the first symptoms being experienced.

There are several stages of dementia, but to classify them properly, the official number according to the global deterioration scale is of 7 stages. We are going to go over all of them, but officially, only 4 of these 7 stages are considered to be dementia.

Stage 1 is when a person is mentally healthy without any kind of issues. This means that they are not being forgetful in any way and they have no problems with their mental abilities at all.

Stage 2

Very mild decline in cognitive functions is found in stage 2, but this is still not considered to be dementia because many people tend to be forgetful and they often misplace items. This is something that a person can start to experience at some point in life but it will never progress to dementia at all.

Stage 3

This is the last stage that is not part of the dementia stages and it means that people might show a slightly higher level of forgetfulness and difficulty focusing and finding the right words to say. This is often due to nutritional deficiencies and stress. It might take about 7 years before this becomes a stage 4 and is classified as early dementia, but it could also stop there and never progress any further.

Stage 4

This is considered to be the first stage of dementia and it's the fourth stage on the list. When a person gets to this stage, they will have more frequent events in which their memory fails them and they will have a harder time managing their finances. They will find it much harder to complete tasks and analyze situations. Once this starts to happen the person might also stop socializing as often and they will experience a harder time managing their social life successfully because their memory loss will become an annoyance to them and to those around them.

Stage 5

This is basically the next level of severity of the same symptoms that have been experienced during stage 4. This means that the frequency of the forgetfulness and difficulty articulating words will be increased.

Stage 6

The severity in this stage is much higher and the patient is no longer going to be able to remember a lot of information about their past. They will start being delusional and their sense of orientation will be badly damaged to the point of needing someone to guide them back to their own homes.

Stage 7

The person is no longer able to control basic body movement and will need to use a wheelchair. Even the most basic activities such as using the bathroom and speaking will become extremely difficult.

17. How to improve healthcare for those affected by Dementia

There is no way to deny that the biggest issue that we are facing right now when it comes to dementia treatment and healthcare, is the lack of awareness of the condition. Everyone has heard of Alzhemier's at this point, but the word dementia is often misinterpreted by people and linked to deranged and violent individuals who are in straightjackets.

Dementia is a very complex disease that will start to attack the brain quite slowly. There are many types of dementia and Alzheimer's is one of them, but the average individual out there has no idea about this and would never associate Alzheimer's with the word dementia. This is mainly due to the lack of proper campaigning to increase the awareness of this terrible illness.

The biggest problem that people with dementia are facing is that healthcare options for this kind of condition are very expensive due to the intensive care that is required when the disease reaches an advanced stage. Some patients might need 24/7 assistance for the last 4 to 6 years of the condition and this is combined with the need for expensive treatments that are often going to require changes in prescription and proper monitoring.

The best way to improve healthcare for dementia is to get more people to see how important it is to find a cure for it. The main hurdle for dementia is that it will never get the level of priority that is given to cancer or heart disease because it's considered to be a disease that only the elderly suffer from. This is true for the most part, but some people are diagnosed with the condition as early as their late 50s and this means their lives are completely halted by the condition.

The future for Alzhemier's treatment is looking good, but there is no cure for this condition at this point. Available treatments help delay the symptoms of brain function deterioration, but the outcome is still inevitably fatal with the current findings and treatments.

If you want to learn how to help support and reinforce the research and healthcare options for this condition, we suggest that you check out all of the available information found here. You can also get involved by being an active contributor in social media. You can post information on dementia and give people important data. This will help them see just how important it is to take proper care of people who suffer from this condition.

18. In search of dementia treatment

There is no question that a search for the cure to dementia is always an important part of the battle between medical science and the conditions that we are unable to cure. Most forms of dementia can be slowed down in order to allow the patient to live for at least 10 to 15 years, but all that has been done with current medicine and treatments is lower the symptom intensity for a few extra years, in order for the person suffering from dementia to be as independent as possible.

The most important aspect of the research for proper dementia treatment is that more people need to contribute to the studies and testing by volunteering to get medical assistance with experimental drugs and treatments. Unfortunately, the very nature of allowing this kind of testing to be done is a huge risk for the patient due to the unknown outcome of those treatments.

The good news is that most of those experimental treatments have allowed doctors to find new treatment options that have been quite successful in slowing down all kinds of dementia, but the idea is to be able to find a cure, or at least slow the progress down at such level that the patient survives the disease by dying of old age before the symptoms become unmanageable.

Increasing awareness of this condition is also going to be very useful and this is going to help determine how much success comes from it. Social media has played a major role in helping raise funds for the cure of dementia and for better treatment options to be given to people who are still in their early senior years and want to be able to live their late years peacefully and calmly.

There is still a lot of road to cover if we are ever to be able to handle this kind of disease. There is nothing more important and valuable than being able to find cures for conditions that have been a burden to humanity since the very beginning, but the truth is that in order to make that happen, we need to make sure that we can get as many people involved and as much funding as possible can be raised for this purpose.

The idea is to be able to eventually reverse and cure the disease and then we will no longer just be looking for ways to slow it down.

19. Stress and how it damages the brain

We live in a society that seems to be perfectly fine with the idea of being stressed out all the time. We feel like we are going to develop a great deal of resistance to the feelings of stress and that we can handle them as often as needed. The problem is that the complete opposite happens with stress. We don't get used to it and we don't develop any kind of resistance to it. Instead, it starts to damage our brain slowly, but steadily.

The constant spikes in our levels of cortisol are going to end up taking a very serious toll on our physical and mental health. There are plenty of studies indicating that chronic stress is highly related to a large number of mental disorders including anxiety, depression and even dementia. This is a serious cause of concern due to how stressful our lives are in modern times and how little time we have to relax and get rid of that stress.

Stress can lead to brain shrinking as it starts to reduce the volume of gray matter inside our brains. The most affected regions are often those that control emotions and physiological functions in general. There is also proof that shows how a very stressful event can lead to brain cell destruction. This means that people who suffer from a great deal of emotionally stressful situations are more likely to end up suffering from a mental condition.

The memory is also going to be highly affected when we are in constant stress. Even worse, the amygdala that is responsible for the processing of fear and fight or flight emotions is constantly triggered even when no serious threat is around and this means that we are in a constant "survival mode" that is taking a very serious toll on our bodies in every possible way.

The best way to avoid this problem is to learn to meditate and to find the time to relax after a hard day of work. A stressful work environment requires that we learn proper time management in order to ensure that we are able to relax after the hard work is over. Exercise, meditate, spend some quality time or even a few laughs with a friend or family member, but whatever you do, you need to make time for your personal relaxation or you will end up with accumulated stress that is very harmful to your health.

20. Understanding signs and symptoms of Alzheimer's disease

Once an individual starts to show signs of mental abilities being lost and difficulty remembering things, this can cause serious concern in the person experiencing those symptoms as well as those around them. The symptoms are noticed by everyone who comes in contact with the person and this means that they will rarely let them go unnoticed or try to hide them because they cannot control when they will show those signs.

It's essential to seek medical attention and get a proper evaluation as early as possible in order to begin proper treatment. This is going to be extremely important because it will give people the time to adjust to the situation and take action. It's very important to understand the signs and symptoms that are often experienced when a person is going through the early stages of Alzheimer's disease.

The mild initial symptoms

The mild symptoms include forgetfulness and having a hard time remembering where you left your car keys and your sunglasses. This is often accompanied by having a harder time expressing thoughts with words and mood changes that happen for no apparent reason. This first stage is usually not going to be too much of a concern until the symptoms worsen and the person seems to be forgetting things quite frequently.

The moderate symptoms

Once Alzheimer's starts to cover more brain tissue, it will start to show moderate symptoms that can become extremely problematic for people. This includes memory loss that makes them forget how to get to places that they have visited frequently and difficulty carrying out tasks as simple as putting on clothes. At this stage, people might even have a hard time recognizing family and friends and it's quite apparent that they are no longer able to function as entirely independent individuals.

The most severe symptoms and stage of Alzheimer's

At this point, all of the symptoms that we have mentioned earlier become even more severe and the person starts to experience problems with the functions of their body. This means they will have a hard time swallowing food and keeping balance. The progression takes about two years from the beginning stages of the severe symptoms until the person is unable to move efficiently and needs to be in bed all day long.

The progression of each stage will depend on the kind of treatment that is given to each person as well as their age and their general health.

21. The survival trends for people with dementia

Just as it happens with the predictions in terms of the incidence of dementia, the survival trends are going to be linked to the number of people who are able to get proper care and the latest medication available to treat the condition. This means that we can predict a higher number of survivors that will manage to die of other old age related conditions while they are receiving treatment for dementia. It's also important to consider the fact that most people will start suffering from dementia at no less than 65 to 70 years of age, so this means that many of them could die of other conditions before dementia is to blame for their passing.

There is no way to deny that we have a large number of diseases to deal with. Some of them have more funding than others and some of them have more support and awareness to back their research up. The important thing to keep in mind is that dementia is a very serious condition that affects a large number of people. The condition slowly deteriorates the brain and many individuals will suffer from it. The condition is emotionally taxing for the patient as well as their loved ones due to how they will eventually even forget who their closest family are and where they live.

The survival trends are looking quite optimistic for developed countries. This is mainly due to the latest medication available, which is extremely expensive for people who are on basic healthcare in their countries or people without insurance. The biggest concern for many of these individuals is that they are likely to have no proper care for their condition and this will cause far faster deterioration of the brain.

It has been proven that the simple idea of being tolerant and understanding with a patient that is suffering from dementia is going to be extremely helpful. Stress has been heavily linked to dementia and once a person is suffering from dementia, higher stress levels are going to contribute to a faster deterioration of the brain.

It seems like developed countries have the advantage of being able to provide better care for people, but the highly stressful modern life is not helping matters even for those who are financially stable. The one factor that is very important in a good economy is that people are more likely to have better dietary habits and to become aware of the need to engage in proper time management to lower stress levels.

22. Understanding Diagnosis and Treatment of Dementia

One of the best ways to help treat any kind of condition is to see what works and what seems to provide no visible results. This means that healthcare facilities need to constantly monitor the quality of life and the progression of each patient with dementia. This needs to be paired up with the kind of experiences that they have with specific medication and treatments that might be enhanced or discarded for future treatments.

The biggest hurdle for dementia care is in the lack of awareness of the condition. Studies show that most people out there don't even know about dementia until someone they know is suffering from the condition. This is not the case with a disease such as cancer because everyone hears about it or knows at least one person who has died of cancer or suffered from it.

One problem with dementia is that proper diagnosis and care for the condition is extremely expensive when compared to other conditions. The process of diagnosis is very tedious and complicated as there are several tests that need to be conducted in order for the condition to be properly diagnosed. This leads to a very frustrating situation for those who don't have insurance that covers this sort of testing.

The social care aspect of dementia is still quite bad in most countries. There are some regions of the world that have proper dementia healthcare facilities that also provide social care and help keep the patients socially active. This is a great way to help them feel happier and to avoid faster mental deterioration due to feelings of frustration and stress.

The treatment coverage needs to branch out and look at people with dementia based on the kind of treatment level they get. There are those who have dementia and have received a conclusive diagnostic. Then you have those who are not diagnosed and still untreated. The other group is those that have been diagnosed but they are not receiving treatment for a number of reasons, and then you have those who have been receiving care since their diagnosis.

Those who have been getting proper care need to be divided between those who are getting acceptable outcomes in the quality of life they have during the condition and those who don't. That is going to reveal what kind of treatment variations work and which ones are not so successful.

23. Assessment & Planning Of Care for those affected by Dementia

Dementia is a very debilitating illness that is not reversible and there is still no cure for it. However, there are ways in which we can help people who suffer from this kind of condition maintain their way of life and that allows them to keep their dignity as much as possible. If certain needs are met, the person affected by dementia is going to be able to live in a safe environment that suits their condition and their limitations.

Proper assessment of the condition is necessary

The treatment for dementia is going to depend on the stage of the condition and how much of the brain has deteriorated because of it. The kind of care that is given to a person on the initial stages of the illness is nothing like the treatment that is given to those who have been suffering from it for a long time.

This is the main reason why the proper evaluation of the condition is essential and tracking its evolution is going to be just as important to make necessary changes in the way that the patient is cared for and treated.

Individual care planning

Every person who suffers from dementia experiences different problems, but most stages have a large number of symptoms that are commonly displayed. With that said, the need for individual care planning is very important and no two patients are going to have the same kind of care given to them.

The process of creating a customized care plan for a patient is going to be determined by their symptoms and their most common reactions when they feel lost or they feel their cognitive skills are failing to help them get through the most common problems.

Family members and friends should be involved

Every person that interacts with the individual that is suffering from dementia should be involved in this process. The ideal situation is for everyone around the patient to know how to deal with any kind of problems and issues that relate to dementia. This is going to create a much better environment for the patient.

Anxiety, depression and a wide range of emotions including anger and indifference are all going to be experienced by people with dementia at some point during the progression of their condition. The best way deal with this is for everyone to be as informed as possible.

24. How can you take care of a person with Dementia?

This is a very common question and the truth is that there is no easy answer for it. There are all kinds of problems that people face when they are dealing with dementia. A caregiver needs to be prepared for several stages that the patient will experience. This is one of the reasons why health care professionals are often trained in dementia care exclusively because this helps them provide the best possible care to their patients.

The first stage

People who are in the first stage of dementia are often going to experience symptoms that they can handle on their own. They are still going to be able to take proper care of themselves during this stage and they will only experience mild memory loss and orientation issues that clear within a few minutes. This is typically a situation that requires no assistance from people, but it would be good for a doctor to start evaluating the patient and keeping track of their progression with the condition.

The second stage

This is going to require assistance because the person is going to start experiencing serious memory loss and they can start to feel lost when driving in the streets and when trying to locate an area that they have visited many times in the past. This is one of the most serious concerns that people experience when they reach this particular stage and that is one of the reasons why it is recommended that they don't go outside without a caregiver or at least with a friend or family member.

This is also a stage that is going to make the person feel extremely frustrated because they won't be able to handle their lack of ability to perform tasks that they once found to be so simple and easy to do. Emotional and psychological support will be very helpful during this stage.

The third stage

This is going to be a difficult stage because the person is no longer going to be able to do anything without assistance. They will lose their independence for the simplest activities and they will need a professional caregiver to help them with everything they need to do.

This is one of the reasons why patients on the later stages of dementia need to be in bed or using a wheelchair most of the time. They can't communicate properly and they even have trouble eating without assistance.

Caring for patients with Alzheimer's is a huge contribution to help those in need while a cure is found for this debilitating and fatal condition.

25. Looking after a patient with dementia

Taking proper care of a person who is suffering from dementia can be a very difficult process. All dementia stages have their own unique set of symptoms and the kind of care that is given to people during those stages is going to depend on the severity of the problem. Some people experience certain symptoms earlier than expected, while others maintain their mental health for longer than most medical records would expect and suggest.

Once a person has reached stage 2 of dementia, they need to be given more attention and someone should be able to keep an eye out on them in case they get seriously disoriented and lost. Once the patient has reached an even higher level and gets to stage 3 of the condition, they will need to be taken care of all day long as even the most basic activities will prove to be impossible for them.

Hobbies and interests

The process of dementia will slowly make the person incapable of working in any kind of profession they once knew, but they can still maintain a good level of interest in hobbies as it is easier to retain that kind of information. This is one of the best things that any caregiver can do in order to help a patient that needs to stay busy and maintain the best possible level of mood and spirits during the progression of the condition.

Get family and friends involved

It's always important for a person who suffers from Alzheimer's to be able to feel as normal as possible. Interacting with friends and family in activities that don't require too much thinking can be a great way to help a patient feel relaxed and experience happiness during those moments. This has been proven to help them slow down the deterioration of their brain.

Taking care of the bedridden

When dementia reaches the final stages, the person is no longer going to be able to stand up, walk, sit, or even hold their own head up straight. This is the stage of the disease that requires attention from a nurse in most cases and the patient will need to be fed and cared for completely.

It's important for patients with dementia to get the help they need and the assistance that will make their illness more bearable as it moves from one stage to another.

26. The importance of palliative care for dementia

Dementia is still a disease without a cure and this makes it an extremely difficult thing to deal with. Proper healthcare for dementia is known as palliative care because what it does is help the patient live with the condition with as much comfort as possible. There are several factors that are needed in order for treatment to qualify as palliative and we are going to go over the basics.

The main goal with palliative care is not to rush or to halt the progress of the condition, but to simply ensure that the person who is suffering from it is going to be able to live the remaining years of their lives without any serious discomfort.

It's also important to establish care planning in order for the patient to be able to let the caregiver know his or her wishes once he condition deteriorates all brain functions and makes it harder for the patient to be able to make decisions as the condition worsens. The best way to handle this kind of situation is to make sure that the patient is able to leave specific instructions of what should be done in regards to their assets and once their mental abilities are no longer optimal.

There should be a formal nomination that gives a person the rights to make financial and personal decisions for the patient in case they didn't leave any specific instructions in any given scenario. This is why it's encouraged for them to make sure that the can provide as much detailed instruction on their wishes before they reach that stage of dementia.

Evaluating the capacity to make decisions

When a person is suffering from a highly debilitating condition such a dementia, they are going to be evaluated by a professional in order to see how their decision-making capacity is doing as the condition moves forward.

In order for someone to qualify as mentally capable, they need to be able to understand all information that is relevant to any decision-making process. They should also be able to retain any kind of information for long enough to make decisions and they should be able to make this decisions without any external influence or coercion.

In conclusion, palliative care and everything that goes along with it is very important for dementia. This is going to help establish a huge difference in the kind of life that people can expect to have when they suffer from dementia.

27. The impact of dementia worldwide in 2015

It can be quite hard to see how little information is out there for those who have never experienced dementia in their social circle. The truth is that never being affected by this disease is just luck of the draw. The statistics on the number of people affected globally is truly alarming and it reminds us of the importance that comes from proper education in regards to this terrible condition. Let's now look at some global statistics that are undeniably relevant and hopefully they will help raise even more awareness on the subject.

In 2015, the number of new cases of dementia all over the world was around 9.9 million. This means that one person every 3.2 seconds was diagnosed with the condition. The biggest concern is that the numbers keep climbing higher every year and there are close to 47 million people living with this condition right now. This number is predicted to increase to 74.7 Million by 2030 and 131.5 Million by 2050 The increase in dementia cases will rise even more in low to middle-income countries due to how much the general wellbeing of an individual is involved in the possibility of having dementia after 65 years of age.

The regions with the lowest number of research facilities that are entirely dedicated to dementia include Africa, Central Asia, Latin America and Eastern Europe. It makes perfect sense that the poorer the country, the harder it is for proper dementia care to be found. This is a condition that is considered to be a disease of the elderly and the priority in developing countries is to use the scarce funds and recourse to treat diseases that attack people of all ages.

There is also an obvious issue with the number of health care professionals that are specialized in the treatment and care for patients that are suffering from dementia. This lack of professional care and the little priority given to the condition makes it even harder for people to get help. There is no estimate time for this to improve in smaller countries, but as long as the economy is in bad shape, the treatment for dementia will remain as a secondary concern.

The incidence of dementia all over the world is considerably large in 2015 and it has been larger than in previous years. The number of people who go onto the internet and search for dementia and Alzheimer's symptoms is also growing all the time.

28. Important facts about dementia in 2016

There are many studies and research campaigns that have been conducted in order to help shine a brighter light on the condition that we know as dementia. We are going to be talking about some of the most important facts that people should know about and how they are affecting the world of dementia care and treatment.

Support for dementia healthcare systems

The first fact to consider is that a smaller level of attention is given to services and centers that are dedicated to the treatment of dementia. This makes perfect sense as there are many other conditions that can be considered more important and relevant for a number of reasons, but the need for more awareness and relevance is huge if we want to see any serious improvements.

Diagnostics coverage

The coverage that is given to proper diagnosis for dementia is quite low. The number of people living with dementia with proper diagnosis for it is as low as 40%. The reason why this happens is because dementia is a very complicated disease that cannot be diagnosed by a single test. There will be blood tests, physical tests and psychological tests that are going to have to be conducted in order for anyone to be successfully diagnosed.

The cost of many of those tests is quite high and this is one of the most compelling reasons why you are very unlikely to see them as part of any basic health coverage plan.

Specialized care is underdeveloped in most countries

There has been an increase in healthcare centers that specialize in dementia treatment, but this is only seen in developed countries. It's very rare to hear of any institution that is specialized in this kind of treatment if the country is experiencing any kind of crisis in the economy. The budgets for medical facilities and staff is usually assigned to conditions that affect a larger number of people of all ages and this kind of priority is logical, but not optimal for the fight against dementia.

Health care funds distribution does not see dementia as a priority. It's hard for a disease that only affects the elderly to become a priority amongst other conditions that are known to affect people of all ages and demographics. The only way to increase funding is to increase awareness so that those who support priority conditions will also consider contributing to the treatment and cure of dementia.

29. Possible trend shifts in the future of dementia incidence

While it can be hard to predict what the immediate or even long-term future is going to be like for dementia, we can already see the possibility of certain things changing. For example, a decline in the incidence of dementia for people between 65 and 70 years of age is a possibility. This is mainly due to a more adequate lifestyle and diet that is the direct result of a social environment that is much more aware of the importance of being healthy and fit.

There are many studies that are leading to the direct relationship between dementia and alcohol or drug abuse. The same goes for tobacco consumption and for poor eating habits. A sedentary life and lack of motivation and drive in life have also become important factors to consider. This is mainly due to the large number of dementia patients that have reported substance abuse of some kind.

Obesity and high cholesterol are also linked to this condition and the number of people with dementia who have at least one of those problems and history of dietary neglect or substance abuse is quite convincing. The one thing that we need to consider is that developing countries are more likely to have a large number of people who have poor dietary habits. The poorer the region, the harder it is for people to consume healthy foods on a daily basis. Also, the lower the economy, the higher the chances that people will engage in drug or alcohol abuse.

These are all factors that could determine the incidence of dementia increasing or decreasing in some regions.

The more developed countries have a lower number of dementia patients when compared to countries that are still developing or currently suffering from a serious financial crisis. Healthcare is extremely scarce in places where more pressing concerns are prioritized.

This is a fact and it will never change. It takes us back to the way society works with everything else. Things that are considered a norm of developed countries are not important or relevant in countries that are facing any serious crisis. If we are to predict the future of dementia incidence, we need to look into the future of each region and country individually for the answers. The best way to ensure a good future is to continue to raise awareness of the condition.

30. The global cost of dementia treatment

The levels of awareness for dementia care and treatment is still quite low when compared to other conditions and diseases. This is to be expected based on the economy of each region, as conditions that only affect the elderly are more likely to be seen as unimportant when compared to other conditions that affect a large demographic. With that said, the global expenses that are related to dementia are on the rise.

The cost has increased from $600 billion in 2010 to $800 billion in 2015. This means that there is an incredibly large number of people who are suffering from the condition and being treated for it. The regional distribution costs for treatment have increased steadily in every region and the need to increase awareness in order to get more support is huge. The global costs of treatment would be fine-tuned if awareness was widespread, but this continues to be such an unknown condition, that most people only know of Alzheimer's and have never even heard of any other form of dementia.

The lower the income in any country, the harder it will be for proper care to ever reach those areas and the available care is extremely expensive for a person with an average job and salary. The prevalence of dementia is going to be determined by a large number of different factors, but the truth is that the countries facing the biggest challenges are the ones that have the lowest income rates.

The costs of dementia treatment are only going to continues to rise all over the world. This will happen as more information is made available on the internet and a larger number of people are diagnosed after they review symptoms online and decide to get checked. Many individuals living with dementia are unaware of the problem until their brain deterioration reaches alarming levels.

The life expectancy of an average individual worldwide is rising, but conditions like dementia are slow acting diseases that could take 10 to 15 years to fully develop into a fatal outcome. This means that the average life expectancy in some regions is 75, but a diagnosis of the condition usually comes between 67 and 70 years of age, which means the person will not die from dementia, but of other health issues. The problem is that it's still very hard to tell just how much of an influence dementia has on other conditions.

CPSIA information can be obtained
at www.ICGtesting.com
Printed in the USA
LVHW040758220122
709106LV00013B/669

9 781543